This report contains the collective views of an international group of experts and does not necessarily represent the decisions or the stated policy of either the World Health Organization, the United Nations Environment Programme, or the International Radiation Protection Association.

Environmental Health Criteria 35

EXTREMELY LOW FREQUENCY (ELF) FIELDS

Published under the joint sponsorship of the United Nations Environment Programme, the World Health Organization, and the International Radiation Protection Association

World Health Organization
Geneva, 1984

ISBN 92 4 154095 8

PRINTED IN FINLAND

84/6131 – VAMMALA – 5500

CONTENTS

Page

Page

NOTE TO READERS OF THE CRITERIA DOCUMENTS

While every effort has been made to present information in the criteria documents as accurately as possible without unduly delaying their publication, mistakes might have occurred and are likely to occur in the future. In the interest of all users of the environmental health criteria documents, readers are kindly requested to communicate any errors found to the Manager of the International Programme on Chemical Safety, World Health Organization, Geneva, Switzerland, in order that they may be included in corrigenda, which will appear in subsequent volumes.

In addition, experts in any particular field dealt with in the criteria documents are kindly requested to make available to the WHO Secretariat any important published information that may have inadvertently been omitted and which may change the evaluation of health risks from exposure to the environmental agent under examination, so that the information may be considered in the event of updating and re-evaluation of the conclusions contained in the criteria documents.

WHO/IRPA TASK GROUP ON EXTREMELY LOW FREQUENCY (ELF) FIELDS

Members

Dr J. Bonnell, Central Electricity Generating Board, London, England

Dr B. Bosnjakovic, Ministry of Housing, Physical Planning, and Environment, Rijswijk, The Netherlands[a]

Dr J. Cabanes, Medical Committee, Electricité de France - Gaz de France, Paris, France

Dr M. Grandolfo, Laboratory of Radiation, Institute of Public Health, Rome, Italy

Dr B. Knave, Research Department, National Board of Occupational Safety and Health, Solna, Sweden

Dr J. Kupfer, Occupational Hygiene Standardization, Central Institute of Occupational Medicine, Berlin, German Democratic Republic (Vice-Chairman)

Dr R. Phillips, Biology Department, Pacific Northwest Laboratory, Richland, Washington, USA

Dr A. Portela, Institute of Biophysical Research, National Council of Scientific and Technical Research (CONICET), Buenos Aires, Argentina

Dr M. Repacholi, Royal Adelaide Hospital, Adelaide, South Australia (Chairman)[a]

Dr A. Sheppard, J.L. Pettis Memorial Hospital, Loma Linda, California, USA (Rapporteur)

IRPA Secretariat

Mrs A. Duchêne, Commissariat à l'Energie Atomique, Déparement de Protection Sanitaire, Fontenay-aux-Roses, France[b]

WHO Secretariat

Mr G. Ozolins, Manager, Environmental Hazards and Food Protection, Division of Environmental Health, WHO, Geneva, Switzerland (Secretary)

Dr M. Shore, National Center for Devices and Radiological Health, Food and Drug Administration, Rockville, Maryland, USA (Temporary Adviser)

---

[a] Members of the International Non-Ionizing Radiation Committee of IRPA.

[b] Scientific Secretary of the International Non-Ionizing Radiation Committee of IRPA.

Electric and magnetic field quantities and units in the SI system

Quantity	Symbol	Unit
Frequency	f	hertz (Hz)
Electric field strength	E	volt per metre (V/m)
Electric flux density	D	coulomb per square metre (C/m^2)
Capacitance	C	farad (F)
Current	I	ampere (A)
Current density	J	ampere per square metre (A/m^2)
Electric charge	Q	coulomb ($C = A \cdot s$)
Impedance	Z	ohm (Ω)
Volume charge density	ρ	coulomb per cubic metre (C/m^3)
Magnetic field strength	H	ampere per metre (A/m)
Magnetic flux density	B	tesla[a] ($1\ T = 1\ Wb/m^2$) (weber per square metre)
Permittivity	ε[b]	farad per metre (F/m)
Permittivity of vacuum	ε_o	$\varepsilon_o = 8.854 \cdot 10^{-12}$ F/m
Permeability	μ	henry per metre (H/m)
Permeability of vacuum	μ_o	$\mu_o = 12.57 \cdot 10^{-7}$ H/m
Time	t	seconds (s)

a 1 T = 10^4 Gauss (G), a unit in the CGS unit system.
b Designates a complex number.

ENVIRONMENTAL HEALTH CRITERIA FOR EXTREMELY LOW FREQUENCY (ELF) FIELDS

Following the recommendations of the United Nations Conference on the Human Environment held in Stockholm in 1972, and in response to a number of World Health Resolutions (WHA23.60, WHA24.47, WHA25.58, WHA26.68), and the recommendation of the Governing Council of the United Nations Environment Programme, (UNEP/GC/10, 3 July 1973), a programme on the integrated assessment of the health effects of environmental pollution was initiated in 1973. The programme, known as the WHO Environmental Health Criteria Programme, has been implemented with the support of the Environment Fund of the United Nations Environment Programme. In 1980, the Environmental Health Criteria Programme was incorporated into the International Programme on Chemical Safety (IPCS). The result of the Environmental Health Criteria Programme is a series of criteria documents.

A joint WHO/IRPA Task Group on Environmental Health Criteria for Extremely Low Frequency Fields met in Geneva from 5 to 9 March 1984. Mr. G. Ozolins, Manager, Environmental Hazards and Food Protection, opened the meeting on behalf of the Director-General. The Task Group reviewed and revised the draft criteria document, made an evaluation of the health risks of exposure to extremely low frequency electromagnetic fields, and considered rationales for the development of human exposure limits.

The International Radiation Protection Association (IRPA) initiated activities concerned with non-ionizing radiation by forming a Working Group on Non-Ionizing Radiation in 1974. This Working Group later became the International Non-Ionizing Radiation Committee (IRPA/INIRC) at the IRPA meeting in Paris in 1977. The IRPA/INIRC reviews the scientific literature on non-ionizing radiation and makes assessments of the health risks of human exposure to such radiation. Based on the Environmental Health Criteria documents developed in conjunction with WHO, the IRPA/INIRC recommends guidelines on exposure limits, drafts codes of safe practice, and works in conjunction with other international organizations to promote safety and standardization in the non-ionizing radiation field.

This document is a combination of drafts prepared by Dr A. Sheppard and Dr W.R. Adey (J.L. Pettis Memorial Veterans Administration Hospital, Loma Linda, California), Dr M.G. Shandala, Dr V. Akimenko and colleagues (A.N. Marzeev Institute of General and Community Hygiene, Kiev, USSR), and Dr P. Czerski and Mr J.C. Villforth (National Center for Devices and Radiological Health, US Department of Health and Human Services, Rockville, Maryland). The drafts were integrated at working group meetings in Grenoble (1980), and Paris (1982). A subsequent draft of the document was prepared by Dr P. Czerski, Dr B. Bosnjaković, Dr M. Repacholi, Dr V. Akimenko, Dr M. Grandolfo, Dr J. Cabanes, and Mrs A. Š. Duchêne at the WHO/IRPA working group in Paris in March 1983. A final draft, incorporating the comments of reviewers from WHO National Focal Points and many international experts, was prepared by Dr M. Repacholi and Dr A. Sheppard in Geneva in December 1983. Scientific editing of the draft, approved by the WHO/IRPA Task Group in March 1984, was completed by Dr M. Repacholi and Dr A. Sheppard. The efforts of all who helped in the preparation and finalization of the document are gratefully acknowledged.

Subjects briefly reviewed, with particular reference to power frequency (50 and 60 Hz) electric fields, include: the physical characteristics of ELF fields; measurement techniques and dosimetry; sources and applications of ELF; levels of exposure from devices in common use; mechanisms of interaction; biological effects in animals and animal tissues; human studies; health risk evaluation and guidance on the development of protective measures such as regulations or safe-use guidelines.

Although the emphasis of this document is on the effects of ELF electric fields at 50 and 60 Hz, effects of ELF magnetic fields are briefly mentioned since they always exist when electric current flows. However, the specific problems related to static and time-varying magnetic fields will be the subject of a separate environmental health criteria document.

Health agencies and regulatory authorities are encouraged to set up and develop programmes to ensure that the lowest exposure occurs with the maximum benefit. It is hoped that this criteria document will provide useful information for the development of national protection measures against ELF fields.

1. SUMMARY AND RECOMMENDATIONS

1.1 Purpose and Scope

This document comprises a review of data on the effects of ELF fields, predominantly ELF electric fields at 50 and 60 Hz, on biological systems pertinent to the evaluation of health risks for man. The purpose of the document is to provide information for health authorities and regulatory agencies on the possible effects of ELF field exposure on human health, and to give guidance on the assessment of risks from occupational and general population exposure. Areas in which uncertainties exist and further research is needed are also indicated.

The document includes a review of the data on the biological effects on human beings and animals of exposure to low frequency electric and magnetic fields in the frequency range of zero to 300 hertz (Hz) (ELF).[a] Data on the biological effects of exposure to sinusoidally varying fields are mainly concerned with effects in the range of 5 - 20 Hz or at 50 and 60 Hz, while limited data are available on effects scattered throughout the ELF spectrum. Data on studies with non-sinusoidal waveforms in this range have also been considered. Effects of electrostatic and magnetostatic fields are not included.

As the document mainly concerns effects directly attributed to ELF electric fields, the effects of co-generated ozone, noise, ultraviolet radiation (UVR) and X-rays from corona discharges, induced short-circuit currents, etc., which may be important factors in the overall transmission line environment, are discussed only briefly.

In general, the effects of contact currents have not been considered in detail since restriction of leakage currents from, for example, household appliances and electromedical devices, is already treated by national and international standards.

1.2 Sources of Exposure

Natural electric fields at extremely low frequencies are very weak, while those of man-made origin are much stronger.

---

[a] According to generally accepted usage in Europe, the region from 30 Hz to 300 Hz is designated as extremely low frequency; the region below this ELF band is unnamed. In the USA, the ELF region is sometimes designated as 0 - 100 Hz (Polk, 1974).

The strongest of the man-made electric fields are those surrounding high voltage transmission lines[a] at 50 or 60 Hz, distribution lines, and traction (transportation) systems that may operate at 16.67, 25, or 30 Hz. Within the home, the proximity of appliances and low voltage wiring produces ambient electric fields of 10^{-1} - 10^{2} volt/metre (V/m), depending on the mains voltage and the distance.

The natural 60 Hz magnetic field is approximately 10^{-9} millitesla (mT), which is low compared with the average fields (up to 0.01 mT) found in private homes. Under the centre line at the midspan of 1100 kV transmission lines, the 60 Hz magnetic field at 1 m above the ground is less than 0.035 mT. This is weaker than the magnetic fields of up to 1 mT that occur close to common household appliances.

It has become common practice to specify fields in terms of their electric and magnetic field strength (E and H). The electric field strength is specified in units of volts per metre (V/m). The magnetic field is given by the field strength H in ampere/metre (A/m) or the magnetic flux density B in weber/square metre (Wb/m^2), where 1 Wb/m^2 = 1 tesla.

1.3 Clinical Applications

The growth of bone tissue can be stimulated by electric currents, and pulsed ELF fields are being used successfully in clinical applications with patients suffering from intractable bone disease or fractures. In the latter technique, electric currents at ELF and higher frequencies are induced by pulsed magnetic fields.

1.4 Field Measurement and Dosimetry

To characterize ELF fields, the strength, frequency, and orientation of the electric and magnetic fields have to be determined. Under power lines, the electric field has its major component oriented vertically (perpendicular to the Earth's surface), while the main magnetic field component is horizontal (parallel to the Earth's surface). Principles of calculation and measurements of these fields are outlined in section 2 of this document.

A human or animal body located in an ELF electric field causes perturbation of the field, resulting in an uneven distribution of the field around the body. Both the electric and magnetic fields induce electric currents in the exposed

---

[a] These fields range up to about 10 kV/m within transmission line corridors, and decrease to a background level of 10^{-4} V/m at approximately 10^{3} m.

body. The electric fields at the body surface and currents induced in man (a biped) and quadruped animals are quite different, even at the same unperturbed field strengths. The factors affecting the magnitude and distribution of fields at the surface of the body and currents induced inside the body are discussed below.

1.5 Characteristics of Biophysical Interactions

In regions of strong alternating electric fields, three interactions occur:

(a) large surface fields exist, particularly at highly curved regions, and may stimulate surface body receptors, producing sensations;

(b) small currents flow within the body due to the large surface fields; their magnitude is very small in comparison with the currents that flow when contact is made with charged conductors. The associated internal electric field is some 10^5 - 10^7 times smaller than the applied external electric field;

(c) spark discharges occur when objects with significantly different potentials approach contact.

In most experimental situations with whole animals or in human studies, the complex interrelationship between surface field effects and possible internal electric field effects makes it impossible to reach a clear conclusion on the importance of each factor.

Although the non-magnetic nature of most biological materials strongly suggests exclusion of magnetic field interactions, alternating magnetic fields can induce electric currents similar to the type of currents induced by coupling to electric fields. However, in the transmission line context, the magnetically-coupled electric currents are generally smaller, but within an order of magnitude of the electric field-coupled currents. For exposures of prolonged duration, currents produced by pulsed magnetic fields (peak intensities of the order of 1 mT) are effective in modifying cell functions (e.g., in the repair of bone fractures in human beings). In laboratory studies with these same fields, changes have been reported in bone growth, amphibian nucleated erythrocyte dedifferentiation, nerve regeneration, and initiation and alteration of DNA transcription, at current densities in fluid bathing body cells of about 1 - 10 $\mu A/cm^2$ and electric gradients of the order of 0.1 - 1 V/m.

The mechanisms by which a weak ELF field may interact with biomolecular systems and tissues are incompletely understood. However, from *in vitro* studies, there is now evidence of field-induced interactions, including the phenomena of ionic interactions with membrane surface macromolecules, which appear to involve coupling of the cell interior to signals from neurotransmitters, hormones, and antibodies.

1.6 In Vitro Studies

In vitro studies are conducted for two main reasons:

(a) to elucidate mechanisms of interaction of ELF fields with biological materials; and

(b) to provide information on end-points to search for *in vivo*.

These studies have included examination of interactions with excised and cultured tissues, cell biochemistry, neurophysiology, and growth of bone tissue. Electric fields were reported to affect endocrine gland secretion, response to hormonal stimulation, brain calcium ion exchange, immunoreactivity of lymphocytes, electrical excitability of neuronal tissue, and tissue growth rates.

Some of these studies have revealed ELF field effects occurring within certain "windows" in frequency and amplitude.

1.7 Experimental Animal Studies

The majority of ELF research has focused on effects directly or indirectly involved with the central nervous system including physiological, ultrastructural, and biochemical alterations, changes in blood composition, behaviour, reproduction, and development. Studies have been conducted almost exclusively on small laboratory animals, except for a few studies carried out with miniature swine and non-human primates.

Although some experimental data exist, one of the most serious shortcomings of the studies on small animals results from an inability to make extrapolations to human beings because of uncertainty about applying the mechanisms proposed for the effects seen so far. In particular, it is difficult to cite equivalent human exposure because of vast differences in the distribution of surface electric field strengths and internal current densities between human beings and animals, and because there are no data on the species dependency of effects.

Studies with small animals exposed to electric fields up to 100 kV/m have revealed effects on components of the nervous system, including synaptic transmission, on circadian rhythms, and on the biochemical properties of brain tissue. Results of behavioural studies suggest that the nervous system may be affected by an ELF electric field that is far too weak to stimulate synaptic function or cell firing, although in vivo studies often do not exclude the possible role of tactile sensory phenomena.

Field effects on peripheral blood composition and biochemistry have been studied by numerous investigators with inconsistent results. Generally, the changes in blood picture involve small deviations from individual norms, but the values usually remain within physiological norms. Results of studies on the influence of ELF fields on immunocompetence in whole animals appear to be negative.

Studies on swine exposed to 30 kV/m and rodents exposed to 65 kV/m for up to 18 months have revealed evidence of teratological effects. These data are not conclusive and do not prove the teratogenic potential of ELF fields in general.

Many studies on genetic effects and effects on cardiovascular function have been reviewed and the conclusion reached that such effects have not been convincingly demonstrated.

1.8 Effects on Man

Existing surveys of the state of health of high voltage (HV) substation workers and HV line maintenance crews have been based on small populations and have produced conflicting results. Soviet authors noted an increased incidence of subjective complaints attributable to effects on the nervous system and shifts in blood biochemistry, but other authors have not reported such observations. Differences in method often make comparison difficult, if not impossible. Field strengths to which personnel were exposed were only estimated, and only approximate data on the duration of exposure to fields in a given strength range were available.

Some studies on volunteers exposed to electric fields up to 20 kV/m for short periods (days), under laboratory conditions, confirmed the existence of slight changes (within the normal physiological range) in populations of peripheral blood cells and biochemistry, similar to those observed in experimental animal studies.

Several recent epidemiological reports have presented preliminary data suggesting an increase in the incidence of cancer among children and adults exposed to magnetic fields through living close to various types of electrical power lines or devices (e.g., power lines coming into the home, transformers, or other electrical wiring configurations), and among workers in electrotechnical occupations.

Slight increases in genetic defects or abnormal pregnancies have been reported in one study. Epidemiological studies have been performed on linemen and switch-yard workers, the groups considered to be subjected to the highest electric-field exposure levels. However, the exposure levels to which these people are subjected have been found to be remarkably low. The preliminary nature of the epidemiological findings, the low levels of exposure, and the relatively small increment in the reported incidence of any effects, suggest that, though the epidemiological data cannot be dismissed, there must be considerable study before they can serve as useful inputs for risk assessment.

No pathological effects resulting from ELF field exposure have been established. However, thresholds for perception, startle, let-go, respiratory tetany, and fibrillation due to contact currents (electric shocks) have been quantified.

1.9 Exposure Standards

The few instances where countries have developed standards limiting human occupational or environmental exposure to ELF fields are discussed and compared in section 9 of the document.

1.10 Conclusions and Recommendations

1. In order to relate biological findings from *in vitro* and *in vivo* studies on experimental animals to human beings, it is recommended that dosimetry studies should be continued to measure and relate external electric field strengths and internal current density distributions in the whole body of both animals and human beings.

2. From studies on man and animals, observed sensitivities are consistent with two proposed models, one on the basis of stimulation of peripheral sensory receptors in strong local electric fields at the body surface, and the other on the basis of current densities induced in the extracellular fluid. It is recommended that models be devised that correlate exposure and biological effects in terms of physical factors, such as surface electric field, tissue current density, spark discharges, and waveform.

3. The continuation of basic research on electric and magnetic field interaction mechanisms is strongly recommended. Investigations should be conducted on the possible synergism or antagonism of field influences with physical and chemical agents, since such data are not available.

4. In some studies, restriction of ELF effects to certain "windows" in frequency and amplitude has been reported. It is recommended that the window concept be further investigated to determine the applicability of data obtained with various frequencies and waveforms, and to relate the findings to potential health detriment in human beings.

5. Studies have been performed on workers with long-term exposure to electric and magnetic fields, but no adverse health effects have been identified. However, these studies were not designed to evaluate effects on reproductive functions, or long-term carcinogenic risks. In two of the studies, electric field exposure was carefully evaluated, and it was found that average exposures in the occupationally-exposed groups were remarkably low.

A suggestion of increased cancer incidence has been reported by a number of investigators who have examined occupational and general population groups exposed to electric and magnetic fields. The studies performed have serious deficiencies in epidemiological design and do not adequately characterize levels and duration of exposure.

The limited knowledge of the potential human health risk associated with exposure to electric and magnetic fields makes it imperative that well-designed epidemiological studies should continue to be undertaken to provide a firmer basis for risk assessment.

6. Occupational exposure to strong electric fields is generally intermittent and of short duration; exposed populations have been identified, and there are some limited data based on practical experience. At field strengths where spark discharges are prevalent, prolonged exposures may impair performance. Such exposures should be avoided, where possible.

7. Linemen working on energized extra- or ultra-high-voltage conductors experience extreme electric field conditions, and the use of appropriate protective clothing or devices is desirable.

8. Whilst it would be prudent in the present state of scientific knowledge not to make unqualified statements about the safety of intermittent exposure to electric fields, there is no need to limit access to regions where the field strength is below about 10 kV/m. Even at this field strength, some individuals may experience uncomfortable secondary physical phenomena such as spark discharge, shocks, or stimulation of the tactile sense.

9. It is not possible from present knowledge to make a definitive statement about the safety or hazard associated with long-term exposure to sinusoidal electric fields in the range of 1 - 10 kV/m. In the absence of specific evidence of particular risk or disease syndromes associated with such exposure, and in view of experimental findings on the biological effects of exposure, it is recommended that efforts be made to limit exposure, particularly for members of the general population, to levels as low as can be reasonably achieved.

10. In principle, electric and magnetic field interference with implanted cardiac pacemakers can lead to reversion to a fixed rate, but cessation of stimulation is possible. Direct interference has not been reported in fields below 2.5 kV/m. Although body currents produced by contact with a vehicle in a weaker field may cause interference, the risk of pacemaker reversion is believed to be slight.

It is recommended that pacemaker designers and manufacturers of other similar electronic equipment ensure that their devices are resistant to failures caused by electric or magnetic field-induced currents.

2. PHYSICAL CHARACTERISTICS, MEASUREMENT, AND DOSIMETRY

2.1 Quantities and Units

The electric (E) and magnetic (H) fields that exist near sources of ELF electromagnetic fields must be considered separately, because the very long wavelengths (thousands of kilometres) characteristic of extremely low frequencies means that measurements are made in the non-radiating near field. The E and H fields do not have the same constant relationship that exists in the far field of a radiating source.

In the vicinity of high-voltage transmission lines, the E and H fields are typically of the order of a few kilovolts per metre (kV/m) and a few tens of amperes per metre (A/m), respectively. Persons standing under HV-transmission lines or in the vicinity of charged conductors will have currents induced in their bodies as a result of the interactions of these fields with the body tissues. To fully assess the health implications of these ELF fields on man, the fields must be measured accurately and interactions with the body described quantitatively. The human body has a complex geometrical structure making it difficult to obtain precise theoretical or experimental descriptions of these interactions.

The quantities and units used in describing ELF electric and magnetic fields are given on page 8.

The electric and magnetic fields are each described by a vector defined by space components along three orthogonal axes. For steady-state sinusoidal fields, each space component can be represented as a phasor, i.e., a complex number having a magnitude and phase. The magnitude is expressed as the root mean square (rms) value of the field strength in volts per metre or amperes per metre, respectively. The electric field strength is defined in terms of a force exerted by the electric field on a unit charge and the magnetic field by the force on a unit current in a unit length of wire.

The flow of charge is the electric current measured in amperes (A). The electric charge is the integral of electric current over time and is expressed in ampere-seconds (A•s) or coulombs (C). Derived quantities are surface charge density ($A{\cdot}s/m^2$) and volume charge density ($A{\cdot}s/m^3$). The current density is defined as the current flowing through a unit area perpendicular to the current direction and is expressed in amperes per square metre (A/m^2).

The electric flux density D is a vector quantity, the divergence of which is equal to the volume charge density. The unit of the electric flux density is $A{\cdot}s/m^2$, and it is related to the electric field strength by the equation D =

εE, ε being the permittivity. Permittivity of the vacuum is $\varepsilon_o = 8.854 \cdot 10^{-12}$ A•s/Vm. The relative permittivity, ε_r, a dimensionless quantity, is defined as $\varepsilon_r = \varepsilon/\varepsilon_o$. In free space, $\varepsilon_r = 1$, but in tissues, the values of ε_r are significantly greater than 1. The capacitance between two objects, measured in farads (1 F = 1 A•s/V), is defined as the charge acquired by an object divided by the potential difference existing between them.

The magnetic field can be described by the magnetic field strength H and by the magnetic flux density B, where $B = \mu H$, μ being the permeability. In free space, $\mu_o = 12.566 \cdot 10^{-7}$ V•s/Am. The relative permeability μ_r, a dimensionless quantity, is defined as $\mu_r = \mu/\mu_o$, $\mu_r = 1$ in air, by definition, and also, for all practical purposes, in biological tissues as well. The magnetic field is an axial vector quantity, the curl (rotation) of which is equal to the total current density, including the displacement current. Magnetic flux density, sometimes called magnetic induction, is expressed in tesla, where $1\ T = 1\ V \cdot s/m^2 = 1\ Wb/m^2$.

When describing exposure conditions, the electric and magnetic field strengths and orientations should be indicated together with the frequency. In the case of AC transmission lines, electric and magnetic field components have a fundamental frequency equal to 60 Hz in North America and 50 Hz elsewhere.

Harmonic content is due to the distortion of sinusoidal waveform of the fundamental frequencies by waveforms of other frequencies, and can be characterized by a Fourier series. The harmonic content may be of importance at points near large industrial loads or in laboratory installations.

Three-phase transmission lines generate fields, the space components of which are not in phase. The field at any point close to line current conductors can be described by the field ellipse, i.e., the field vector describes an ellipse in any full cycle. At distances of about 15 m or more away from the outer conductor, the electric field of transmission lines can be considered practically a single phase field.

The vertical component of the electric field under a transmission line is the rms value of the component of the electric field along the line perpendicular to the ground and passing through the point of measurement. This quantity is often used to characterize induction effects in objects close to ground level.

The space potential of a point is a phasor representing the voltage difference between the point and the ground. The space potential is perturbed by the introduction of an object into the field. The "unperturbed space potential" that would exist if the object were removed is often used in describing the field. This is the induction field potential.

It is important to consider the action of an electric field on the human body. Within the body, the low frequency electric field is attenuated by about 10^5 - 10^7 from the value of the external field. This is in contrast with a magnetic field. Because of the high conductivity of the human body, the electric field is distorted and localized at the surface of the body. In an alternating field, a current is produced within the body, that has the same frequency as the external field.

The human body acts as a conductor at ground potential, when a person is in good electrical contact with earth, as when wearing conducting shoes. A person wearing well-insulated shoes assumes a free or floating potential above ground. However, the resistance to earth of a person wearing shoes with leather soles is about 15 kΩ and with plastic shoes about 100 MΩ (Deno, 1977). When the body is earthed, a current flows through the body to ground. This current is approximately 14 μA (for 50 Hz) and 17 μA (for 60 Hz) for each 1 kV/m of undisturbed field strength (depending on the body size and shape). Of this current, about one-third flows into the head (Hauf, 1982).

Kaune & Gillis (1981) formalized a number of concepts that simplify the description of the interaction between an animal and an ELF electric field. These authors showed that the electric-field intensity at the surface of the body and induced currents passing through various segments of the body are determined by: (a) the characteristics of the applied electric field, i.e., field strength, spatial structure, and frequency; (b) the shape of the body; (c) the location of the body relative to ground and other conductors; and (d) any conduction currents from the body to ground or other conductors. Because these quantities do not depend on the internal structures of the body, they can be measured using conducting models, which may be hollow. The authors showed that the electric field outside the body and the induced charge density on the surface of the body are independent of frequency in the ELF range for both grounded and ungrounded exposure conditions. They also showed that the electric field outside and inside a body will be unchanged by a scaled change in the size of the body. Finally, these authors proved that the electric charge induced inside the body of an exposed human being or animal is small compared with that induced on the surface of the body.

The magnetic field is not perturbed by objects that are free of magnetic materials. Magnetic field induction in objects causes two types of electric currents (Zaffanella & Deno, 1978):

- a circulating current inside the object (eddy current) induced by the magnetic flux density; and
- a current entering and leaving the object which may be induced by the magnetic flux density through some large loop external to, but including, the object.

2.2 Computational Methods and Measurements of ELF Electric Fields

Computational methods for the determination of electric and magnetic fields are presented in standard textbooks on engineering and physics. Detailed data on computational methods for in case of HV transmission lines are presented in The Transmission Line Reference Book (1975) and Zaffanella & Deno (1978).

There are basically two different approaches to the measurement of 50 or 60 Hz E fields:

(a) free-body probes that measure fields at points remote from the ground (Transmission Line Reference Book, 1975; Bracken 1976); and

(b) ground-reference instruments that measure the current to ground that is collected by a metallic surface (Miller, 1967).

The principles of operation of both types of instruments are closely related. A free-body instrument consists of a hollow metallic shell that is cut in half and the two halves insulated from each other. The displacement current intercepted by a half-shell is the time derivative of the surface unit charge, and for a sinusoidal field:

$$I = dQ/dt = k\omega\varepsilon_o E \cos\omega t \qquad \text{Equation (1)}$$

where E is the E-field strength, Q is the charge induced on one of the half-shells, ω is the angular frequency, ε_o is the permitivity of free space, and k is a constant.

The theory of operation for the ground-reference instrument is quite similar to the above. A flat reference plate is placed on the ground in electrical contact with the ground. A second plate is placed a small distance above the reference plate and insulated from it. The displacement current is again given by Equation (1).

The free-body approach is recommended for outdoor measurements near power lines, since it does not require a known ground reference for measurements anywhere above ground. The ground-reference probes can be used only under special conditions as discussed in the Transmission Line Reference Book (1975).

The electric field is perturbed (in some circumstances significantly) by the presence of human beings, vegetation, or other structures. Data presented in the literature show that, as a general rule, in the presence of each perturbing influence, the measured values are somewhat less than the unperturbed ones.

Three main procedures are used for the calibration of E-field instruments:

(a) parallel plate techniques (usually with guard rings);
(b) single ground plate;
(c) current injection (Miller, 1967).

These three techniques have been reviewed by Kotter & Misakian (1977). The first method is the best as it provides an accuracy of 1% or better for calibration of the field.

The electric field strength meter should be calibrated periodically at intervals determined by the stability of the meter. The instrument on a long (at least 2.5 m) handle is held between the plates at the centre of the structure to take the appropriate measurements while the plates are at a known voltage.

For some instruments, a correction for temperature and humidity may be required. Therefore, these parameters should always be recorded at the time of calibration and at the time measurements are made.

In 1978, IEEE presented a technique using parallel plates to calibrate power-line field survey meters. Two parallel, square metallic plates separated by a distance d are supplied by an alternating voltage source. The electric field strength E at the midplane of the setting is given by:

$$E = V/d$$

where V is the voltage difference existing between the plates. Fringing field effects at the periphery of the plates tend to modify the field that would be expected to occur at the centre point of the plates. It was found that for a pair of parallel plates 1 m^2 each and spaced 0.5 m apart, the variation in field magnitude was less than 1% from the simply computed value at the centre in the midplane. This system constitutes a simple method of evaluating survey meters.

For additional data, see the IEEE Standard for Recommended Practices for the Measurements of Electric and Magnetic Fields from Power Lines (IEEE 1978, 1979) and Tell (1983).

2.3 Field Polarization and Homogeneity

At ground level, beneath the transmission line, the electric field is essentially a vertical homogeneous field with a horizontal component that is about 20% of the vertical component (Poznaniak et al., 1979). At distances of more than 15 m from the outer conductor, this horizontal field drops to less than 10% of that of the vertical field (Zaffanella & Deno, 1978).

Most experimental arrangements for the exposure of animals involve a pair of horizontal parallel electrodes to produce a vertical electric field that is quite homogeneous, if the electrode spacing is adequate. Calculations (Ware, 1975; Shih & DiPlacido, 1980) indicate that the unperturbed electric field strength between parallel plates is quite uniform in both the horizontal and vertical directions, when the horizontal dimensions are two or more times greater than the distance between the plates.

2.4 Energy Carried by the Field

A 10 kV/m electric field has an energy density of $4.42 \cdot 10^{-4}$ J/m^3 producing an average power density in the body of man of about 10 μW/m^3, which is about 10^{-8} times the metabolic rate of the human body (Sheppard & Eisenbud, 1977). Thus heating of a body by an ELF field is completely negligible.

2.5 Determination of ELF Field Exposure

There are no universally accepted and clearly defined concepts relating ELF field "dose" to biological effects, comparable with ionizing or radiofrequency dosimetry in terms of exposure and absorbed doses. Deno (1977), for example, suggests that exposure to the electric field can be expressed as the product of electric field strength and the duration of exposure. The current dose (charge) on the various body surfaces and inside the body is a constant ratio in the unperturbed field, if a person stays erect. An "equivalent" E field is the vertical field at ground level (0.5 m), which would cause the same induction space potential at each body position. The fields induced inside the body depend only on the charges at the body surface (Deno 1979).

A "dose monitor" to measure the electric field exposure in terms of the time integral of the unperturbed field in the ranges of 0 - 5 kV/m, 5 - 10 kV/m, and above 10 kV/m has been constructed. A separate device discharges the integrator monitors and gives a reading of the doses after the exposure period. The actual exposures were shown to be lower than those obtained by multiplying the electric field strength in the area of work by the total time spent in these areas. A similar device, constructed by Lövstrand et al. (1979), was used to measure the exposure of workers in 50 Hz EHV-substations. Lövstrand et al. (1979) stressed, however, that the relationship between the unperturbed electric field strength and the biological effect was by no means clearly established. They maintained that further work was needed to develop dosimetric concepts and to establish the relative significance of surface charge densities, internal electric field strength, current, and current densities for the "dose"-biological effect relationship.

2.6 The Physical Interaction of Man and Laboratory Animals with Electric Fields

The exposure of intact organisms to ELF electric fields is conventionally specified in terms of the unperturbed field strength, in V/m or kV/m, which is measured or calculated before the subject enters the field. The unperturbed field is not, however, the field that acts directly on an exposed subject. The fields to which a subject is actually exposed can be categorized as follows:

(a) Electric fields acting on the outer surface of the body. These fields can cause hairs to vibrate and can thereby be perceived; they may also be able to stimulate other sensory receptors in the skin.

(b) Electric fields induced inside the body. These fields act at the level of the living cell, and their presence is accompanied by electric currents because of the conductivity of living tissues.

It has been shown that electric fields at the surface of a conducting object are enhanced relative to the unperturbed field, while induced fields inside the body are attenuated by about 10^6 (Barnes et al., 1967; Deno, 1977; Kaune & Phillips, 1980).

2.6.1 Surface fields and internal current density

The electric field lines (the directions along which a charge is moved by the force imposed by the field) are perpendicular to the surface of the body. A greater concentration of electric field lines (i.e., higher field strength) exists at a curved surface, such as the human head, than on less curved surfaces of the body. For this reason, it is useful to specify the surface electric field that exists on various parts of the body.

A conducting object placed in an electric field carries a current that is directly related to these surface fields. Thus, the internal currents are greatest at the areas of the most intense surface electric field. The current carried within the body (or a portion thereof) can be calculated from the capacitance of the body, a quantity that takes into account the size and shape of the body and its proximity to other conducting objects such as the ground and high voltage electrodes or wires, or perhaps other animals, fences, trees, etc. (Deno, 1974, 1975, 1976, 1977; Bracken, 1976; Zaffanella & Deno, 1978; Kaune & Phillips, 1980).

Within the body, the two quantities of interest are the current and the current density. The total current is more easily measured or calculated, but the current density is more directly relevant in discussion of electric field effects in a particular tissue or organ. The electrical complexity of the interior of the human body, due to the presence of insulating membranes and tissues of various impedances, has so far frustrated confident analysis of precise interior current densities (Kaune & Phillips, 1980; Spiegel, 1981).

2.6.2 Capacitive coupling of the electric field to man and laboratory animals

A body is coupled to an electric field in proportion to its capacitance such that the greater the capacitance the greater the current flow in the body. For example, the capacitance of a rat is about 5 picofarad (pF), while human beings have capacitances of about 125 pF, when in close proximity with ground (Deno, 1974; Deno & Zaffanella, 1975).

In many laboratory exposures of small animals, the distance between the animal and the lower electrode is small or nonexistent so that the animal's capacitance to this lower (usually earthed) electrode represents a substantial portion of the total capacitance.

By definition, in capacitive coupling, the body, according to its capacitance C, "acquires" a certain amount of surface charge Q and attains a potential $V = Q/C$. This view finds formal expression in models that express any arbitrarily complex body as an equivalent plate at an equivalent height, such that the total current collected by the plate is the same as that for the actual body (Deno, 1974). The capacitance, and thus the induced current, decrease for a body separated from the ground and not close to the energized electrode. The capacitance is dependent on the size, especially on the surface area, shape, and orientation of the body, so that internal currents will differ between fat and thin persons, between persons standing and reclining, and between persons walking barefoot and those wearing thick rubber-soled shoes or standing on a platform. It would be useful, in all cases, to define the conditions under which the capacitance has been measured.

A short-circuit current I_{sc} flows in a body placed in an electric field and connected to the ground through a low resistance path (paws, bare feet, a hand grasping an earthed pole). This current is the sum of all the displacement currents collected over the surface of the body. The only place on the body where a current of the magnitude of the short-circuit current flows is where there is connection with the ground.

2.6.3 Shock currents

In contrast with capacitive coupling to the field, a person touching a conductor carries a "shock current", the magnitude of which is determined by the total circuit impedance including the electrical impedance of the skin and body. Exposure to an extremely strong electric field would be needed to produce displacement currents of several milliamperes, which would represent a hazard similar to that of touching a live wire (Schwan, 1977).

2.7 Dosimetry and Scaling Between Laboratory Animals and Man

The surface and induced fields to which quadrupeds (e.g., laboratory animals) and bipeds (e.g., human beings) are exposed are markedly different at the same unperturbed field strength. Hence, it is necessary to scale exposures across species to compare biological responses.

At present, there are several ways in which electric-field exposure effects found in animals might be scaled to possible effects in human beings. One way is to scale on the basis of equivalent surface electric fields. Alternatively, the induced currents or electric fields in corresponding tissues and organs could be determined.

When scaling of exposure is made on the basis of equivalent surface electric fields, it is assumed that the mechanism by which biological effects are produced involves stimulation of receptors on the surface of the body or currents at the surface of the body. Stimulation of peripheral somatosensory receptors has been demonstrated by Jaffe (1982, in press). Also, electric fields at the surface of the body can produce oscillation of hairs on the surface with a resultant stimulatory effect.

Classical neurophysiology suggests that induced current densities could produce changes in cell physiology when transmembrane current densities are of the order of 0.1 mA/cm² (Schwan, 1982b). Large current densities are not normally possible because such high E fields would be needed that electrical breakdown of the air would occur long before these current densities could be induced. Novel mechanisms of interaction of the E field with various biological systems would be needed to explain any effects at the current densities of 10^{-6} - 10^{-9} A/cm² that may be caused by fields found in the environment.

An erect grounded human being (biped) couples more strongly to an ELF electric field than laboratory animals (quadrupeds). Surface electric fields and axial current densities have been measured in models of man, pig, and rat by Kaune & Phillips (1980) (Fig. 1). At the tops of the bodies, surface electric fields are enhanced over the unperturbed field strength present before the subjects entered the field by factors of 18, 6.7, and 3.7 for human beings, swine, and rats, respectively. For an unperturbed field strength of 10 kV/m, average induced axial current densities in the neck, chest, abdomen, and lower part of the legs are, respectively: 550, 190, 250, and 2000 nA/cm² for human beings; 40, 13, 20, and 1100 nA/cm² for swine; and 28, 16, 2, and 1400 nA/cm² for rats.

Recently an attempt has been made to determine human exposure conditions simulated by animal exposures to 60-Hz electric fields (Guy et al., 1982). A thermographic method for determining the specific absorption rate (SAR) was used to quantify the electric current distributions in homogeneous models of animals and human beings exposed to uniform 60-Hz electric fields by exposing models (of scaled size and conductivity) to 57.3 MHz fields. Although the values of maximum current density predicted in the ankles of models of human beings exposed to 60-Hz fields at 1 kV/m, 200 nA/cm, agreed with independent measurements on full-scale models, the simulation of the 60-Hz field with a 57.3-MHz field may not be exact, when determining corresponding current densities in animals and man.

Theoretical models of biological effects of electric fields must distinguish between the importance of the microscopic electric field versus the microscopic electric current, although these two quantities will always be interrelated. If the model for interaction depends on transport of a certain quantity of charge, then the microscopic electric field is not the quantity of interest, and various experimental results should be scaled according to

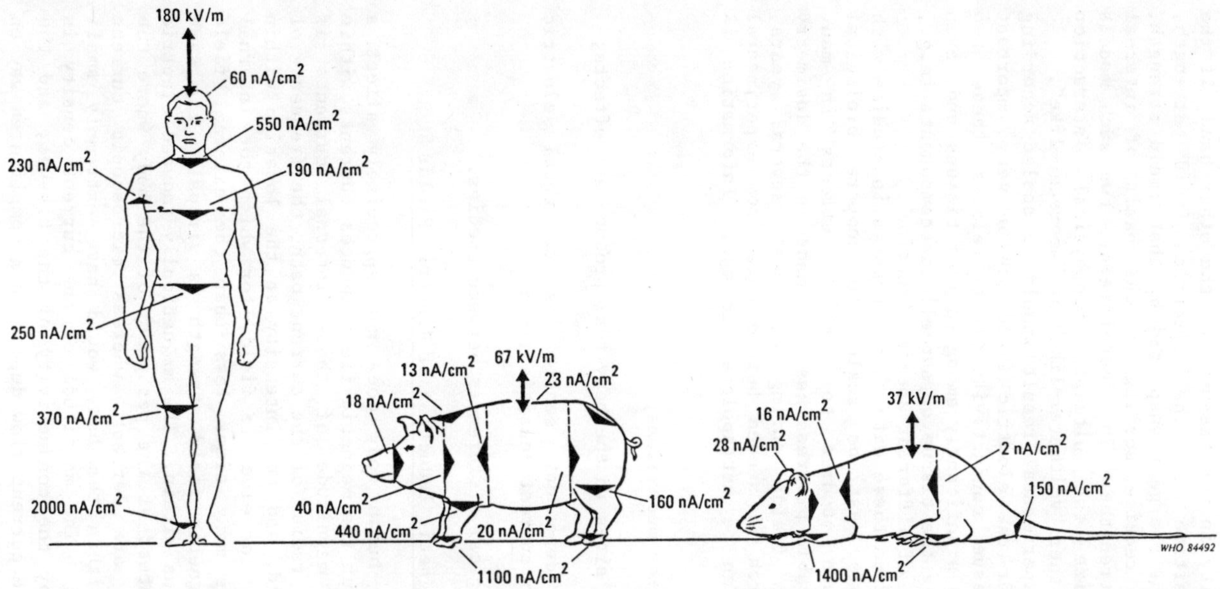

Fig. 1. Grounded man, pig, and rat exposed to vertical, 60-Hz, 10-kV/m electric field. Relative body sizes are not to scale. Surface electric field measurements for man and pig and surface field estimates for rats are shown. Estimated axial current densities averaged over selected sections through bodies are shown. Calculated current densities perpendicular to the surface of body are shown for man and pig (From: Kaune & Phillips, 1980).

the current density in the tissue. On the other hand, if the tissue is sensitive to the electric field strength, independent of the charge transported by that field strength, the model would require scaling on the basis of internal electric field strengths. In general terms, two such models would characterize the ultimate biophysical interaction measurement as either "voltmeter-like" or "ampmeter-like".

Whether an experimental result should be scaled according to the current or the electric field can be very important because the tissue conductivity that relates these two quantities varies signficantly among various tissues and, even more widely, among the tissue or subcellular components (e.g., plasma membranes) of different species (section 5).

It is clear from these data that exposures in studies with laboratory animals must be scaled to compare biological effects from such studies to possible effects in man. Although considerable progress has been made in the dosimetry of ELF electric fields during the past several years, additional research is needed before data from experimental animal studies can be extrapolated to man. Information is needed on:

(a) interaction mechanisms;

(b) critical sites in the body that produce any effects;

(c) species dependent sensitivies to equal electric fields or current densities; and

(d) physiological differences between species.

2.8 Magnetic Induction of Electric Fields

An animal or human body does not appreciably affect a magnetic field, but the magnetic field induces currents within the body. The magnitude of these internal currents is determined by the radius of the current path, the frequency of the magnetic field, and its intensity at the location within the body. Unlike the electric field, for which the internal field strength is many times less than the external field strength, the magnetic field strength is virtually the same outside the body as within. The magnetically-induced electric currents are greatest at the periphery of the body where the conducting paths are largest, whereas microscopic current loops anywhere within the body would have extremely small current densities. The magnitude of the current density is also influenced by the conductivity of the tissues, and the exact paths of the current flow depend in a complicated way on the conducting properties of tissues.

The induced current density and power absorbed by a prolate spheroid model of a man exposed to the magnetic-field component of a transmission line have been calculated by Spiegel (1977).

3. NATURAL BACKGROUND AND MAN-MADE ELF FIELDS

3.1 Natural Electric Fields

The electric and magnetic fields of the Earth consist of a static component, which is dominant, and a time-varying component, which is smaller than the static component by several orders of magnitude in the 50 - 60 Hz frequency range (Polk, 1974). The fields are characterized by vertical components E_z and H_z for the electric and the magnetic fields, respectively, as well as by two horizontal components $E_{x,y}$ and $H_{x,y}$.

The most important sources of man-made fields in the ELF range operate at the power frequencies of 50 Hz or 60 Hz. The natural electric field strength at the power frequencies of 50 Hz or 60 Hz is about 10^{-4} V/m, which means that fields in the close vicinity of HV transmission lines are 10^8 times stronger, and the fields introduced into homes by wiring or appliances are still about 10^3 - 10^6 times stronger than the natural background.

The natural electric field near the Earth's surface is a static field of about 130 V/m (Dolezalek, 1979). This is due to a separation of electric charge between the atmosphere and the ground, so that the Earth resembles a spherical capacitor and the ground and upper atmosphere represent conducting surfaces. Daily changes in the natural electric field are attributed to factors, such as thunderstorms, that affect the rate of charge transfer between the ground and the upper atmosphere. According to Chalmers (1967), thunderstorms have electric fields of 3 - 20 kV/m.

The alternating fields at low frequency are related to thunderstorm activity and magnetic pulsations that produce currents within the Earth (telluric currents). The strength of the Earth's electric field varies in time and over the frequency range 0.001 - 5 Hz (Krasnogorskaja & Remizov, 1975). Local variations occur depending on atmospheric conditions and variations in the magnetic field. The main characteristic of the Earth's electric field are presented in Table 1.

3.2 Natural Magnetic Fields

The natural magnetic field is composed of an internal field, due to the Earth acting as a permanent magnet, and to an external magnetic field in the environment from such components as solar activity, telluric currents, atmospheric activity, etc.

Table 1. Characteristics of the Earth's electric field in the ELF range

Frequency range (Hz)	Nature of the field	Field strength (V/m)	Reference
0.001 - 5	Short duration pulses (magnetohydrodynamic origin)	0.2 - 1000 for E_z	Krasnogorskaja & Remizov (1975); Vanjan (1975)
7.5 - 8.4 and 26 - 27	3 - 6 quasisinusoidal pulses of undetermined origin during an interval of 0.04 - 1 s	On the average, (0.15 - 0.6) 10^{-6} for $E_{x,y}$ with a maximum of 10^{-6}	Beresnev et al. (1976)
5 - 1000	Related to atmospheric changes (atmospherics) present all the time	10^{-4} - 0.5 for E_z, and one order of magnitude lower for $E_{x,y}$. The amplitude decreases with increasing frequency	Aleksandrov et al. (1972); Presman (1971); Kleinmenova (1963)

The internal magnetic field of the Earth originates from the electric current in the upper layer of the Earth's core. There are significant local differences in the strength of this field, varying from about 50 A/m at the poles to about 23 A/m at the equator (Presman, 1971; Benkova, 1975). These field strengths also vary with time.

The external magnetic field consists of many components differing in spectral and energy characteristics (Aleksandrov et al., 1972; Polk, 1974; Benkova, 1975). The variations in the magnetic fields are related to solar activity, particularly with respect to the ELF components, which change over 11-year and 27-day periods and also exhibit circadian variations. Other causes of variations in the natural magnetic fields are thunderstorms, atmospheric changes, and air ionization. About 2000 thunderstorms are occurring simultaneously over the globe, and lightning is striking the Earth's surface about 160 times per second; the currents involved may reach $2 \cdot 10^5$ A at the level of the Earth (Kleimenova, 1963). Electromagnetic fields having a very broad frequency range (from a few Hz up to a few MHz), originate the moment lightning strikes and propagate over long distances, influencing the magnitude of magnetic fields.

The characteristics of the Earth's magnetic field can be summarized as follows:

(a) The amplitudes from $4 \cdot 10^{-2}$ to $8 \cdot 10^{-2}$ A/m are at pulsation frequencies ranging from 0.002 to 0.1 Hz.

(b) The geomagnetic pulsations up to 5 Hz are of short duration, lasting from a few min to a few h.

(c) The amplitude of the field decreases with increasing frequency from $8 \cdot 10^{-6}$ A/m at 5 - 7 Hz to $8 \cdot 10^{-9}$ at 3 kHz.

(d) At 50 or 60 Hz, the natural magnetic field is approximately 10^{-9} mT (Polk, 1974).

The geomagnetic field exhibits temporal and spatial variations related predominantly to solar activity and local magnetic aberrations.

3.3 Man-Made Sources of ELF

3.3.1 High-voltage transmission lines

The principal man-made sources of ELF are HV transmission lines, and all devices containing current-carrying wire, including equipment and appliances in industry and in the home operating at power frequencies of 50 Hz in most countries and at 60 Hz in North America.

Electrical energy is transmitted from the power plant, where it is generated, along conductive, metallic transmission connections (overhead power lines or underground cables) to substations and finally to energy consumers.

A typical overhead line (Fig. 2) consists of supporting structures (transmission towers or pylons) from which the live conductors are suspended by sets of insulators. Each set of insulators supports a single conductor or a bundle of two or more conductors, which carries one electrical phase of the power supply. The conductors of each phase are suspended far enough away from the other conductors and the transmission tower to prevent flashover or short-circuiting between one phase and another, or between the phases and earth (via the supporting structure). In overhead lines, the conductors consist of bare metal cables. Thus, any approach to a live conductor presents a lethal danger due to flashover and a resulting electric current flow that would precede actual contact with a conductor.

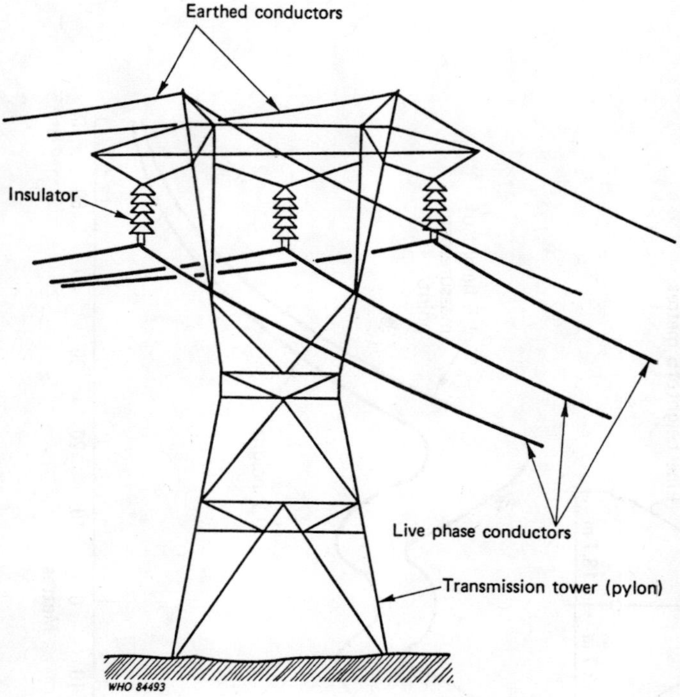

Fig. 2. The basic structure of a single circuit 3-phase power line.

High voltage lines are operated at standard voltages up to 750 or 765 kV and a line at 1100 kV is operating in the USSR. The construction of 1000 - 1200 kV or 1500 kV lines is in progress or at various stages in planning.

Most widely used are alternating current (AC) 3-phase HV lines. One circuit of the 3-phase line comprises 3 single or 3 sets of conductors under high-voltage and 1 or 2 grounded conductors that protect the live conductors against lightning.

Typically, the unperturbed electric field at the height of an average man, standing at the location of the maximum field (just outside the outer conductor) of a high-voltage transmission line of 750 kV, is of the order of 10 kV/m. A lower value of about 1 kV/m exists where the line is highest from the ground (20 m) and about 12 kV/m where it is lowest (13 m) (Zaffanella & Deno, 1978). The electric field strength is a function of the lateral distance from the centre of the HV line as shown in Fig. 3.

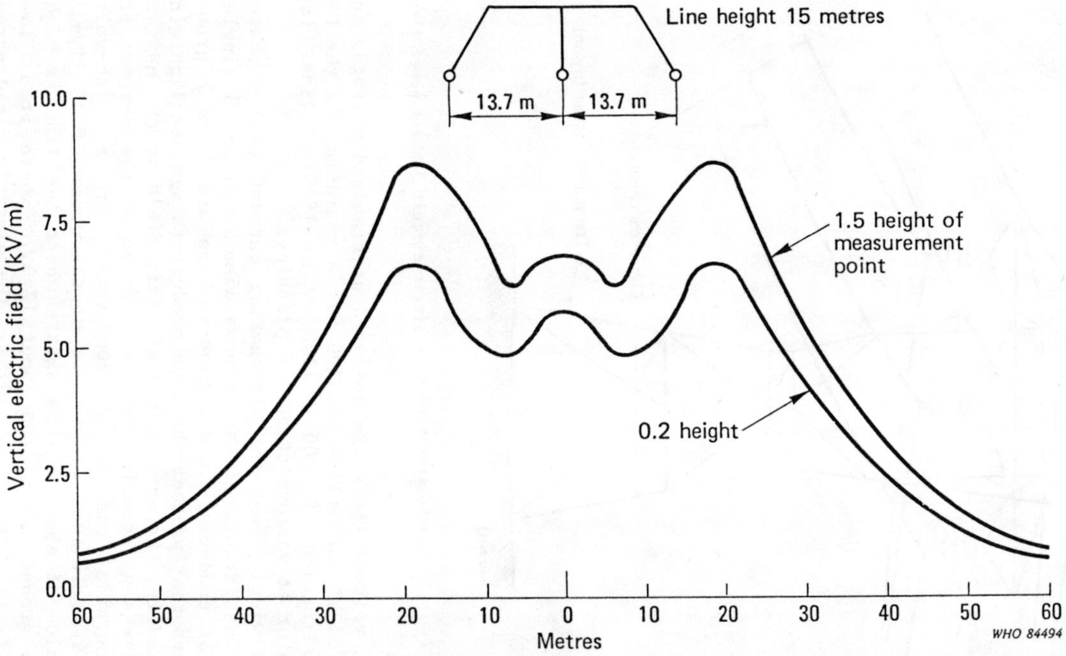

Fig. 3. Unperturbed electric field measured under a 765-kV 60-Hz transmission line (From: Bridges, 1975).

Occupational exposures that occur near high voltage transmission lines depend on the worker's location either on the ground, or at the conductor during live-line work at high potential. When working under live-line conditions, protective clothing may be used to reduce the electric field strength and current density in the body to values similar to those that would occur for work on the ground. Protective clothing does not weaken the influence of the magnetic field.

3.3.2 Electric fields near transmission lines and substations

At ground level, beneath high-voltage transmission lines, the electric fields created have the same frequencies as those carried by the power lines. The characteristics of these fields depend on the line voltage, and on the geometrical dimensions and positions of the conductors of the transmission line. The field intensity selected for reference or comparison purposes is the undisturbed ground level electric field strength. To avoid the effects of vegetation or irregularities in the terrain, the unperturbed field strength is usually computed or measured at a given height above ground level (0.5, 1, 1.5, or 1.8 m).

There are several primary influences on the electric field strength beneath an overhead transmission line. These include:

(a) the height of the conductors above ground (which is influenced considerably by the ambient temperature and heating caused by the current passing through the conductor);

(b) the geometric configuration of conductors and earthing wires on the towers, and in the case of two circuits in proximity, the relative phase sequencing;

(c) the proximity of the grounded metallic structure of the tower;

(d) the proximity of other tall objects (trees, fences, etc.);

(e) the lateral distance from the centre line of the transmission line;

(f) the height above ground at the point of measurement; and

(g) the actual (rather than the nominal) voltage on the line.

Inside buildings near HV transmission lines, the field strengths are typically lower than the unperturbed field by a factor of about 10 - 100, depending on the structure of the building and the type of materials (Manders & van Nielen, 1981).

Conductor height, geometric configuration, lateral distance from the line, and the voltage of the transmission line are by far the most significant factors in considering the maximum electric field strength at ground level. At lateral distances of about twice the line height, electric field strength decreases with distance in an approximately linear fashion. Reference to typical measured or calculated field contours in the vicinity of the line (Zaffanella & Deno, 1978) indicates that, for a 525 kV transmission line (height about 10 m), the field is always less than 1 kV/m at distances of more than 40 m from the outer conductor, while for a 1050 kV line, which has much higher conductors, the 1 kV/m field occurs at a distance of about 100 m from the outer conductor. Typically, where a right-of-way (Row) is used for a transmission line of 500 kV or more, it varies from 35 to 70 m, so that electric fields at the edge of the RoW are of the order of 1 kV/m.

The electric field strengths at and above ground level from various transmission lines are shown in Fig. 4 (Gary, 1976). The electric field distribution within various voltage substations is given in CIGRE (1980).

3.3.3 Magnetic fields near transmission lines

Just as an electric field is always linked with the presence of charges, a magnetic field always appears when electric current flows. A static magnetic field is formed in the case of direct current, whereas time-varying electric and magnetic fields are induced in the vicinity of alternating current power transmission systems.

The magnetic field beneath high-voltage overhead transmission lines is directed mainly transversely to the line axis. The maximum flux density at ground level may be either on the route centre line or approximately under the outer conductors, depending on the phase relationship between the conductors.

Apart from the geometry of the conductor, the maximum magnetic field strength is determined only by the magnitude of the current. The maximum magnetic flux density at ground level for the most common overhead transmission line systems is approximately 0.1 mT/kA (Hylten-Cavalius, 1975).

In contrast to an electric field, a magnetic field is more penetrating and very difficult to shield. It easily penetrates human beings and, in the case of an alternating or

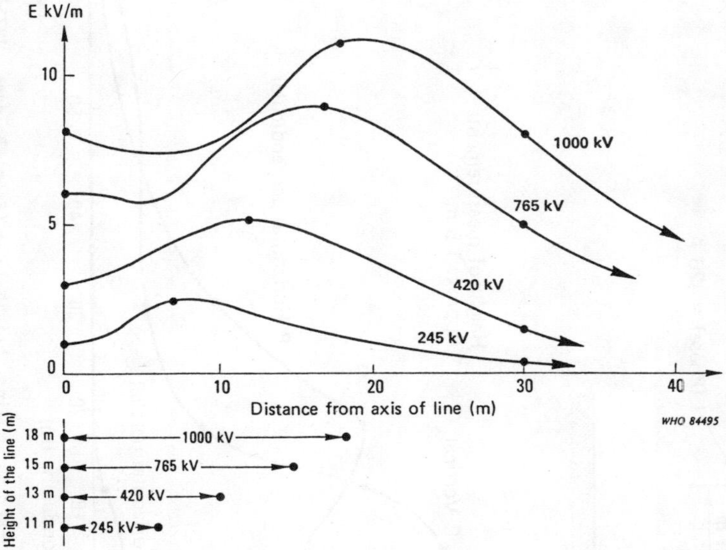

Fig. 4. Values of electric field strength at end above ground for various voltage transmission lines (From: Gary, 1976).

rotating field, induces circulating or eddy currents that are not conducted to ground. The internal voltage differences induced within the body by a magnetic field from power lines may be as high as 1 mV, if the magnetic flux density reaches approximately 0.028 mT (Hauf, 1982).

The maximum ground level magnetic field strengths associated with overhead transmission lines are of the order of 0.01 - 0.05 mT and are also related to line height. Unlike the electric field, they are also directly affected by the current carried by the line. The magnetic flux density decreases in an approximately linear fashion with distance from the conductor (Lambdin, 1978; Zaffanella & Deno, 1978).

In principle, these magnetic fields can induce electric currents in the body and could induce effects via the same mechanisms as electric field-produced currents. However, for exposures near a HV transmission line, the smaller magnitude of these magnetically-induced currents (generally no more than 25% of the electric field-induced currents) has resulted in little emphasis on their contribution. The largest current densities occur at the periphery of the body and they are lower inside. Fig. 5 and 6 show the magnetic field

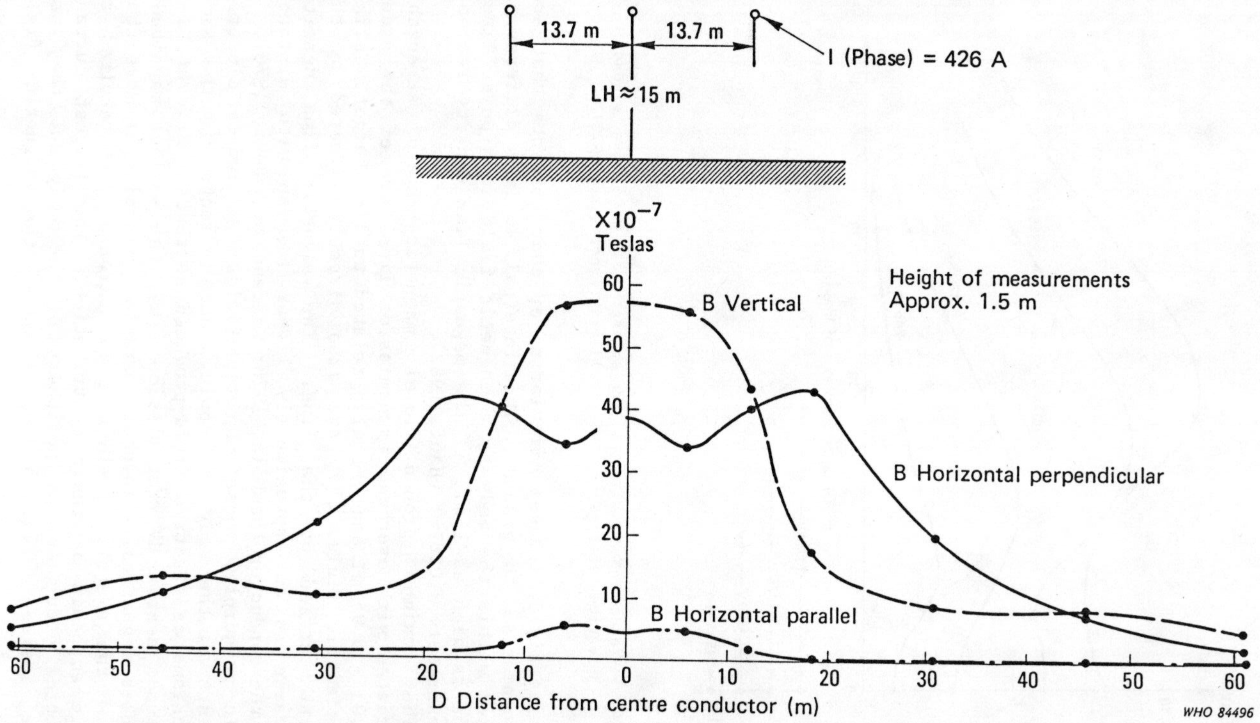

Fig. 5. Profile of three magnetic field components under a 765-kV, 60-Hz line, height 15 m (From: Bridges, 1975). Components of B are shown for orientations in the vartical plane and in horizontal planes for directions parallel or perpendicular to the length of the line. Current load is about 10% of maximum.

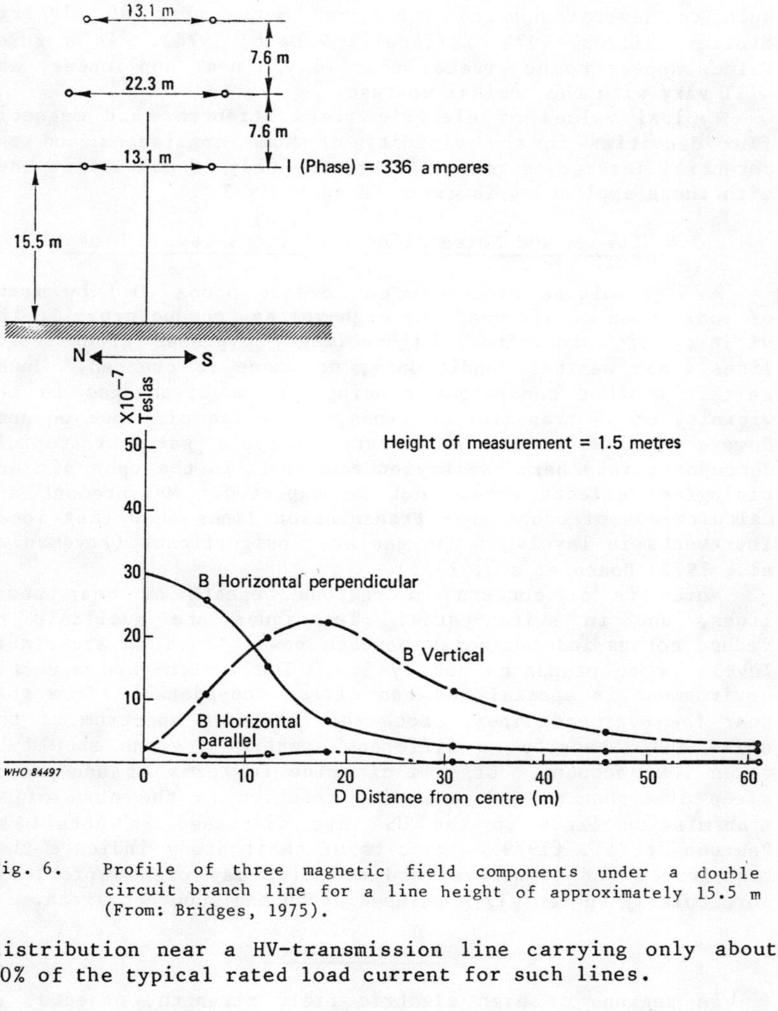

Fig. 6. Profile of three magnetic field components under a double circuit branch line for a line height of approximately 15.5 m (From: Bridges, 1975).

distribution near a HV-transmission line carrying only about 10% of the typical rated load current for such lines.

3.3.4 Man-Made ELF Fields in the Home, Workplace, and Public Premises

In the home or workplace, ELF electric field sources occur at electric wiring, appliances, and light fixtures, or industrial electrical machines. Measurements of electric fields in a typical American home (115 V circuits) ranged from less than 1 V/m to about 10 V/m, while fields measured at 30 cm from some appliances varied from 2 to 5 V/m near a light bulb to several hundred volts per metre near an electric broiler (Miller, 1974; Zaffanella & Deno, 1978). As a rule, values appear to be greater than 10 V/m near appliances, and will vary with the nominal voltage.

Typical values of electric field strengths and magnetic flux densities in the vicinity of home appliances and the potential leakage currents through the body if contact is made with these appliances is given in Appendix I.

3.4 Corona and Noise Effects of Transmission Lines

A high-voltage electrode can create ozone (O_3) by means of ionization of air near the high-voltage conductors. In the vicinity of corona-free, high-voltage, overhead transmission lines (fair weather conditions), no ozone is created. Under certain weather conditions causing corona discharges in the vicinity of HV transmission lines, formation of ozone occurs. However, since ozone is a very unstable gas, it rapidly decomposes into harmless oxygen compounds in the open air and biological effects should not be expected. Measurement and calculations of ozone near transmission lines show that local increments in levels of the gas are insignificant (Frydman et al., 1972; Roach et al., 1973).

Noise is of concern in regions beneath or near power lines, and in switch-yards. Techniques are available to reduce corona-induced noise beneath power lines to acceptable levels or to standards set by law. The switch-yard acoustic environment is special and can differ considerably from that near the overhead lines. Both the frequency spectrum of the noise and intensity in different spectral regions should be taken into account. Effects of noise in terms of annoyance, sleep disturbance, and community reaction in the case of HV transmission lines in the USA are discussed in detail by Pearsons et al. (1979). Results of their study indicate that transformer and transmission line noise may create problems, particularly in densely-populated urban and suburban areas.

3.5 Electric Shock

In regions of high electric field strength, objects, if insulated from ground, can assume large potential differences. If the human body becomes the pathway for currents between such objects, substantial electric currents (of the order of 1 mA) can flow. Investigation of these effects has revealed two exemplary cases in which significant shock currents exist:

(a) a long unearthed metal fence running parallel to the line; and

(b) a large vehicle beneath the conductors and effectively insulated from ground.

It is necessary to distinguish between the transient short-circuit current and the steady-state short-circuit current. Zaffanella & Deno (1978) presented data, obtained under various circumstances, that indicated that peak currents of up to 20 A can flow for a few microseconds when a person draws a spark discharge from an object with a hand-held metal key. The peak currents are an order of magnitude smaller if the finger is used for contact. The energy content of spark discharges obtained from a carpet are found to be similar to those in a 10 kV/m electric field with the important exception that the AC field continually recharges the electrified body so that repeated frequent sparks are possible, whereas several steps must be taken on a carpet to recharge the body. The steady-state short-circuit current that flows when the charged object is earthed depends on the capacitance to earth of the object, and the open-circuit voltage to which the object is charged, when disconnected from ground, according to the relation: $I_{sc} = \omega V_{oc}.C$, where I_{sc} is the short circuit current, ω is the angular frequency of the electric field, V_{oc} is the open circuit voltage, and C the capacitance to earth of the object (Deno, 1974).

For human beings standing on the ground with arms at the side of the body in an electric field of frequency f, the short circuit current I_{sc} in amperes is given approximately by the empirical formula (Deno, 1974):

$$I_{sc} = 9.0 \cdot 10^{-11} h^2 E \cdot f$$

where f is 50 or 60 Hz, h is the person's height in metres (m), and E the electric field strength in volts per metre (V/m). Thus, in a 10 kV/m, 60 Hz electric field, a person 1.7 m tall carries a short circuit of about 160 μA.

Typical capacitances for objects range from 700 pF for a small vehicle to several thousand pF for buses and large trucks and about 1000 pF for a 150 m fence (Deno, 1974). Thus, the short-circuit current for a 150 m fence could be as great as 2.2 mA, if the fence were located in a field of 5 kV/m. Zaffanella & Deno (1978) measured the short-circuit currents of a farm tractor, jeep wagon, and a school bus. In a 10 kV/m electric field, these vehicles conducted 0.6, 1.1, and 3.9 mA of current to earth, respectively. Although the shock currents are of appreciable magnitude, they should not present a hazard if appropriate safety procedures are followed. Good engineering practice to reduce the risk of shocks includes the carefully earthing of fences, gutters, and other long metallic objects in a strong electric field.

Data (Zaffanella & Deno, 1978) concerning human beings exposed to spark discharges of various intensities showed that 50% of the population perceived spark discharges in a field of 2.7 kV/m and that 50% of the population found the spark discharges annoying at 7 kV/m. To obtain these data, persons standing in an electric field touched a metallic post with a finger; it is assumed that their capacitance was of the order of 170 pF.

The sensations that result from microshocks do not appear hazardous (except insofar as they may produce a startle reflex that could result in an accident), but they may be highly significant in the evaluation of effects attributed to the fields. Although the scope of this document does not include the possible health effects of such microshocks or transient spark discharges, more than cursory mention is given to these effects because of their importance.

For the human responses, it is useful to define 3 thresholds:

(1) Perception: the minimum current for perception by touch is about 0.4 µA;

(2) the Let-Go Current: the maximum current for which a person can release the involuntary muscular contraction (Fig. 7) (Dalziel & Lee, 1968);

(3) the Fibrillation Threshold: the minimum body-current to cause ventricular fibrillation is especially dependent on the pathway of the current in the body and the duration (Fig. 8) (Kupfer, 1979; Kupfer et al. 1981). If the current is directly applied to the heart, the fibrillation threshold is about $5 \cdot 10^2$ times lower (Kupfer, 1982; Weirich et al., 1983).

3.6 Interference of ELF Fields with Implanted Cardiac Pacemakers

An implanted pacemaker is an electromedical device that artificially stimulates the heart, thus making it possible for persons with certain heart diseases to lead relatively normal lives. Although pacemakers may be susceptible to some forms of electrical interference, hazardous situations resulting from ambient electromagnetic fields have not been reported. Results of a research programme reported by Bridges & Frazier (1979), who carried out bench studies and studies with implants in animals, showed a wide range in interference sensitivity among various devices and for different arrangements of the implanted leads.

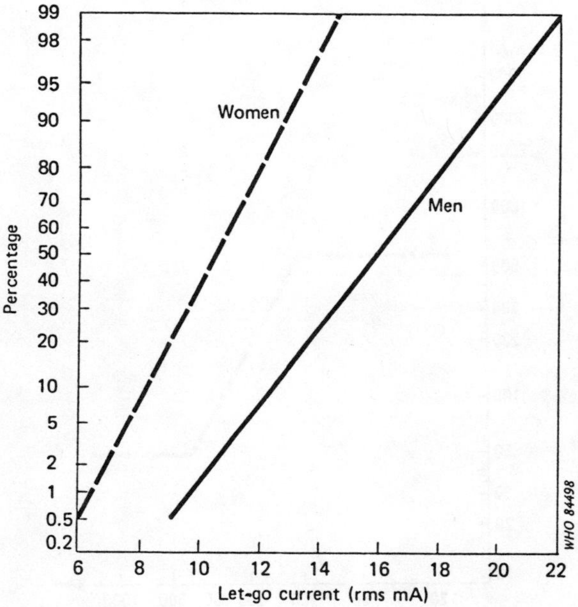

Fig. 7. Let-go current threshold distribution for adults, 60-Hz current (Adapted from: Dalziel & Lee, 1968).

Pacemaker reversion can be brought about via the following three mechanisms (Bridges & Frazier, 1979):

(a) direct coupling to an ambient electric field (typical threshold range, 3 - 600 kV/m);

(b) transient coupling to an ambient electric field through vehicle leakage current ("microshock") (typical threshold range, 60 V/m - 60 kV/m);

(c) coupling to appliances having a leakage current (typical threshold range, 40 - 6000 μA).

Butrous et al. (1983) studied 35 patients (fitted with 16 different pacemaker models from 6 manufacturers) who were exposed to 50-Hz electric fields up to a maximum of 20 kV/m. Current flow measures varied between 15 and 300 μA, depending on the field strength and the position of the patient in the field. Four different response patterns were encountered: (a) normal sensing and pacing in all conditions (one manufacturer); (b) reversion to the fixed (interference)

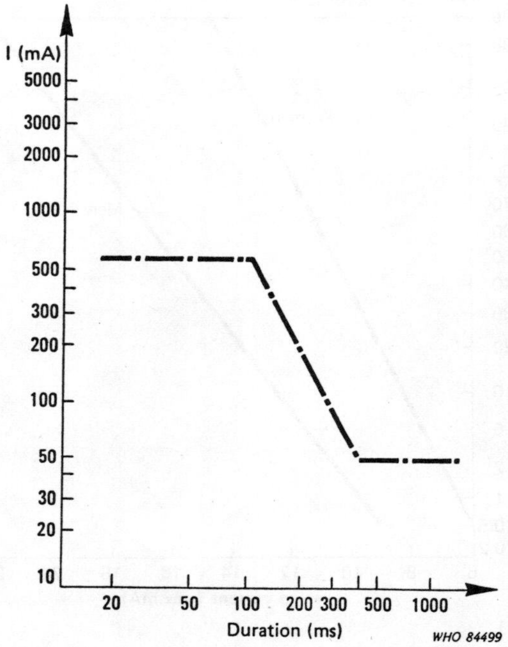

Fig. 8. Proposed maximum allowed body current I (mA) and duration (ms) in human beings to be safe from ventricular fibrillation (From: Kupfer et al., 1981).

rate; (c) slow and irregular pacing; and (d) mixed behaviour over a critical range of field strengths and then reversion to a fixed rate. Their responses depended on the pacemaker units. The field strengths required to induce such behaviour varied with unit and model. Generally, the interference threshold depended on the magnitude and distribution of induced body current relative to the pacemaker, as well as field strength, and thus varied with patient height, build, and posture.

4. MECHANISMS OF INTERACTION

Several mechanisms have been proposed to explain the reported effects of ELF electric fields on laboratory animals, and in tissues and cells *in vitro* including:

a) stimulation of peripheral receptors in the skin;

b) induced electric fields and currents inside the body acting at the level of cells; and

c) non-specific stress.

4.1 Biophysical Mechanisms of Electric Field Interactions

Electric field coupling occurs through capacitive and conductive modes. Energy is transferred to the object from the E field and an electric charge in the object is put into motion. The amount of charge involved depends on the size and location of the object with respect to the E field. When a path to ground is provided, the charge movement results in a current flow. If the object is insulated from the ground, a potential develops with respect to the ground, the magnitude of which depends on the capacitance to ground.

The penetration depth of the field lines into the body is very shallow at low frequencies. There is evidence that the field induces direct effects on skin sensors of the cat paw at a threshold local field strength of over 200 kV/m (Jaffe, in press). Some reported behavioural effects in chickens, mice, rats, and pigs exposed to unperturbed fields of 30 - 100 kV/m may be related to sensory stimulation. These effects are presented in reports on field perception, arousal, avoidance, transitory activity changes, and transitory increases in cortecosterone levels (Moos, 1964; Graves et. al., 1978; Hjeresen et. al., 1980; Sagan et. al., 1981; Rosenberg et. al., 1983; Stern et. al., 1983).

With large field strengths, discharges may be detected. Small currents flow within the body due to capacitive coupling to the fields. In principle, an electric field of sufficient magnitude could have a direct effect on biological tissues by acting directly on the free ions in the extracellular milieu, on the charged portions of the biomolecules, or by interaction with electric moments of molecular electronic structure. However, the very small internal electric fields that result from capacitive or magnetic coupling (Barnes et al., 1967; Sheppard & Eisenbud, 1977) could not affect covalent molecular structures or the electrostatic bonds between molecules, nor could there be direct effects on steric structure.

In his consideration of ELF electric field interactions with neural cells, Schwan (1977) stated that, under a wide range of assumptions for cellular shape and cellular electrical properties, it was impossible that the largest electric fields in air could significantly affect neural membrane potentials by the passage of transmembrane currents. Schwan added, however, that the anomalous properties at frequencies below 100 Hz, though still poorly understood, "provide for more possibilities of subtle effects if there are any at all".

Adey (1980) suggested that it is important to take into account the possibility that one cell may influence another in brain and other tissues through modulation of their shared electrochemical environment. The same author (Adey, 1981) proposed that amplification of the weak initial stimulus occurs by a cascade of intracellular processes taking place at receptor sites on the cell membrane surface. This model may be supported by data on the coupling of the parathyroid hormone receptors to the cyclic adenylase and cyclic AMP responses in bone cells (Luben et al., 1982).

It was suggested by Cain (1981) that voltage-sensitive ion channels play a role at sufficiently large field strengths. He proposed that an alternating potential across the cell membrane may change membrane conductance by interacting with the charged groups of the protein macromolecules that gate voltage-sensitive ion channels.

Pilla (1980) developed a model for electrochemical information transfer at membrane surfaces that involves a minimal electrostatic perturbation of the molecular structure. The essence of the model is that specific surface adsorption is expected to exhibit a significantly longer relaxation time than dielectric or electrostatic interactions, due to the number of aqueous and membrane steps involved, so that the characteristic time for adsorption may be about 10 ms. This is in agreement with data obtained from toad bladder membrane (Pilla & Margules, 1977). This mechanism would work in parallel with the charge transfer processes already known to occur, and could mediate enzymatic reactions to have significant effects on cellular chemistry.

Recently, Schwan (1982a,b) discussed the possible role of alternating field-induced ponderomotoric forces, i.e., forces exerted by electric fields on nonpolar particles. The theory developed on this basis can be used to explain dielectrophoresis (Pohl, 1978), rotation, deformation, destruction of cells (Schwan, 1982a), and electrical cell fusion (Pilwat et al., 1981; Richter et al., 1981) in cases where electric field strength greatly exceeds that which could be produced in tissue by an environmental ELF field.

4.2 Biophysical Mechanisms of Magnetic Field Interactions

The eddy currents created by magnetic ELF fields in the human body cannot be measured directly, but they can be calculated and confirmed by measurements on phantom models. The biological effects of such induced electric currents are discussed above, but any direct magnetic field effects are not well understood at present.

5. BIOLOGICAL EFFECTS IN CELLS AND ANIMALS

Since human volunteers cannot be used for studies that could potentially cause harmful effects, biological investigations are normally conducted using various other animal species. Studies have been performed, mainly using rats and mice, but a wide variety of other subjects, including insects, birds, dogs, swine, and non-human primates, have also been used. A broad range of exposure levels have been employed, and an equally large number of biological end-points have been examined for evidence of possible electric-field effects. Since all animal studies cannot be discussed, this review will be limited to studies having some bearing on health risk assessment. Experiments not discussed will be summarized in the tables. Some studies showed effects from exposure, and others showed no effects. There is general consensus among scientists that exposure to electric fields produces biological effects; however, more data are still needed to determine whether these effects constitute a hazard.

Many studies have been performed based on the explicit or implied hypothesis that because electrochemical processes are involved in nervous system functioning, there might be an interaction of the electric field with the nervous system. Such hypotheses became of greater interest when initial reports on linemen and switch-yard workers (Asanova & Rakov, 1966; Korobkova et al., 1972) suggested the occurrence of a generalized alteration in central nervous system function. Other studies were based on generalized physiological hypotheses, such as the expectation that electric field exposure, continued over a long period of time, might induce a stress response, alter cardiovascular function, affect immune responses, or alter various biochemical and physiological variables, especially blood chemistry and blood cell populations. Study areas briefly reviewed below also include growth and development, reproduction, fertility, and behaviour.

Studies on the effects of electric and magnetic fields on the ecosystems involving plants, invertebrates (including insects), birds, fish, and mammals have been summarized (Lee et al., 1979, 1982). As these studies do not have a direct relevance for human health risk assessment they are not discussed further.

5.1 Cellular and Membrane Studies

The effects of electric fields on *in vitro* systems have been studied in a few laboratories. With these studies, it is possible to use large sample sizes and to have a high degree of control over experimental variables. Such studies also provide a more direct investigation of the possible mechanisms of interaction between a biological system and an electric field. However, the most serious problems with in vitro experiments are those of dosimetry and extrapolation. The dosimetric relationship between exposure in cellular systems and in whole animals is unclear, and extrapolation of results from less complicated systems to human beings is extremely uncertain.

Preliminary experiments using cultured Chinese hamster ovary (CHO) cells exposed to 3.7 V/m showed no effects on cell survival, growth, or mutation rate (Frazier et al., 1982). Cell-plating efficiency, however (reflecting a possible alteration in the cell membrane), was reduced in cells exposed to 60-Hz fields at strengths greater than 0.7 V/m. At the same field strength (0.7 V/m) (Marron et al., 1975; Goodman et al., 1976, 1979), after several months of exposure, slime mold showed frequency-dependent effects on mitotic rate, cell respiration, and protoplasmic streaming. These effects were observed with both electric fields and magnetic fields, alone or in combination.

Studies using a variety of models (Greenebaum et al., 1979a,b; Miller et al., 1979) have given contradictory results. Effects on cell division, growth, and metabolism may appear at field strengths of the order of tenths of a V/m or tenths of a mT in the medium. On the other hand, electrical cell rotation and fusion (Pohl, 1978) appear in the range of 10 - 100 kV/m.

Experimental findings suggest that the principal site of interaction between ELF fields and the interior of living systems is the cell membrane (Adey, 1975, 1977, 1980, 1981; Bawin et al., 1975, 1978; Sheppard & Adey, 1979; Adey et al., 1981). These include a 10 - 20% alteration in the calcium exchange from chick or cat brain tissues exposed to ELF electric fields, either amplitude-modulated radiofrequency (RF) carrier waves of 50, 147, or 450 MHz, or ELF sine wave fields (Bawin et al., 1975, 1978; Blackman et al., 1979, 1980, 1982). The calcium effect is windowed in frequency, where maximal effects occur for 16 Hz modulation, and in the case of direct ELF exposures, Blackman et al. reported several windows at 15 Hz and its harmonics up to 105 Hz, in fields of less than 100 V/m in air. A similar narrow amplitude window limits the range in field strength (Bawin et al., 1978; Blackman et al., 1979, 1982). Bawin et al. (1978) found a relationship between the observed effect and the ionic composition of the bathing medium.

In the case of the ELF modulation of a RF field, the magnitude of the effective ELF field (obtained by demodulation of the RF field envelope) that acts on the calcium-binding sites depends on an unknown efficiency for a demodulation process occurring at an unidentified site. Assuming complete demodulation, the effective ELF field would correspond to an ELF-only field in air of the order of 100 kV/m (Adey, 1981), though by use of the RF carrier there is no significant heating of tissue (Tenforde, 1980) and no known artifact (such as spark discharges).

A calcium efflux effect is also reported for in vivo studies on the cat (Adey, 1980). Possible underlying biophysical mechanisms and a relationship to the electric properties of the brain (electroencephalograph waves or EEG waves) are discussed by Grodsky (1976). However, the physiological implication of the calcium efflux phenomenon is not known.

Electric field effects on synaptic transmission and peripheral nerve function in rats exposed for 30 days to a 60 Hz field of effective strength 65 kV/m were studied in replicate (Jaffe et al., 1980, 1981). The exposure apparatus was designed to eliminate the confounding influence of electric shock currents. Neurons of the superior cervical ganglion showed significantly increased excitability compared with the control group, as determined from tests in which the amplitudes of paired compound action potentials were measured (conditioning test response or C-T response). None of several other indices of neural function was altered to a significant extent. The authors interpreted the data as evidence of an effect on pre- or post-synaptic mechanisms, possibly indicating enhanced excitability, and as evidence against a significant effect on nerve conduction mechanisms.

An investigation (Wachtel, 1979) in which invertebrate neurons from the sea hare Aplysia were exposed in vitro to a low-frequency electric field indicated a strong frequency dependence in response to extracellular currents that included synchronization with the applied field. The neuron was most sensitive at frequencies below 1 Hz, close to the natural firing rate of Aplysia neurons, and for a particular neuronal orientation with respect to the field. Other data were reported by Sheppard et al. (1980) concerning the ELF field exposure of Aplysia neurons, including transient changes in the firing rate and increased variability during exposure to an electric field of 0.25 V/m rms. Episodic synchronization between the neuron and the applied field was reported at $1.4 \cdot 10^{-4}$ A/cm² (rms).

In a study by Bawin et al. (in press) on rat brain tissue slices exposed to either 5- or 60-Hz electric fields at field strengths in the range of the EEG, 1 - 10 V/m, evidence was presented of long-lasting changes in neuronal excitability that differed with field frequency and exposure duration. While 5-Hz fields were generally excitatory, brief 60-Hz fields either potentiated or depressed the tissue response following field exposure, and prolonged 60-Hz fields depressed the response. Although potentiations (believed to be due to an effect on synaptic mechanisms) can last indefinitely (observations have lasted for as long as 7 h), the depressed response after 60-Hz exposures was transient, lasting about 10 min.

In summary, the results of in vitro studies suggest that time-varying ELF electric fields may change the properties of cell membranes and modify cell function. Several theoretical explanations have been proposed (section 4), and it seems conceivable that several parallel mechanisms exist. No comprehensive and experimentally confirmed theory has been proposed. Some of the effects observed on cells and tissues in vitro can be detected in vivo.

5.2 Neurophysiological Studies in Animals and Animal Tissues

Blanchi et al. (1973) reported changes in the electroencephalograph (EEG) patterns of guinea-pigs exposed for 30 min to a 100-kV/m, 50-Hz electric field. Gavalas et al. (1970) noted EEG spectral power peaks in the hippocampus, and less frequently in the amygdala and centrum medianum, in all three monkeys exposed in 7- and 10-Hz electric fields (7 V/m peak to peak). Others failed to see any EEG alterations in chicks exposed at 40 kV/m (Bankoske et al., 1976), and cats exposed at 80 kV/m (Silney, 1979). EEG effects have not been reported in other studies.

Hansson (1981a,b) reported that Purkinje cells of the cerebella of rabbits exposed to the 14-kV/m (50-Hz) field of an outdoor substation or exposed in the laboratory showed pathological changes in the cellular cytoskeleton and alterations in the concentrations of two glial cell proteins (S-100, GFA). When young rabbits were exposed to a 50-kV/m electric field for 6 months, no ultrastructural changes were found in cerebellar cells, nor changes in several plasma hormones (Portet & et al., 1984).

Jaffe et al. (1981) found a significant effect of field exposure (30 days, 65 kV/m) on neuromuscular physiology for one type of muscle (slow-twitch soleus), but not for another (fast-twitch soleus).

The data from neurophysiological tests in vivo and in vitro indicate that electric fields may have effects on tissues, especially components of the nervous system. The physiological significance for human beings exposed to environmental fields has not been determined. Information is needed on the relationships between biophysical and biological effects. In some in vitro studies, the fields or current densities clearly exceed the values estimated for internal fields or current densities in human beings exposed to environmental fields.

5.3 Behavioural Studies

Among the most sensitive measures of insult to a biological system are tests that determine modifications in the behavioural patterns of animals. This sensitivity is especially valuable in studying environmental agents of relatively low toxicity (Anderson & Phillips, 1984). Behavioural studies in several species provide evidence of field perception and the possibility that the fields may directly alter behaviour. In rats, the threshold of detection varies from subject to subject in the range of 4 - 10 kV/m with an average level at about 8 kV/m (Sagan et al., 1981; Stern et al., 1983). In mice, responses to a 35-kV/m field were reported (Rosenberg et al., 1983); perception was seen in pigeons at approximately 30 - 35 kV/m (Graves, 1977), and in pigs at 30 - 35 kV/m (Kaune et al., 1978).

Hjeresen et al. (1980) reported on field avoidance among rats exposed at 75 - 100 kV/m (60 Hz). Preference for shielded areas at night was found among pigs exposed at 30 kV/m (Hjeresen et al., 1982). However, at 25 kV/m, rats preferred the field region during the inactive phase (Hjeresen et al., 1980). Tests of aversion in rats exposed to fields of 32 - 130 kV/m produced a complex pattern of null effects in some cases (Creim et al., 1980) or positive effects in others (Lovely, 1982), depending on the behavioural test.

Alterations in rat activity were noted at 1.2 kV/m by Moos (1964). Other studies on activity indicated transitory increased response on initial exposure of rats or mice at 25 - 35 kV/m (Hjeresen et al., 1980; Rosenberg et al., 1983), depressed activity in chickens exposed at 26 - 40 kV/m (Bankoske et al., 1976; Graves et al., 1978), and increased activity among bees exposed at 4.2 kV/m (Greenberg & Bindokas, 1981).

Tests with monkeys at 7 - 100 V/m exposed to frequencies typical of the EEG (1 - 32 Hz) showed altered behavioural reponses in an operant conditioning task (Gavalas et al., 1970; Gavalas- Medici & Day-Magdaleno, 1976), while in other tests involving exposure to magnetic and electric fields, behaviour was unaffected (DeLorge, 1972, 1973). Feldstone et al. (1980) observed minor changes in behaviour among baboons exposed to 30 kV/m (60 Hz).

Tests on the behaviour of cats exposed to ELF-modulated radiofrequency signals were reported to show evidence of long-lasting, frequency-specific changes in brain rhythms (EEG), and studies of brain rhythms in rabbits exposed to

ELF-modulated radiofrequencies were also reported to show specific changes in the EEG (Takashima et al. 1979).

Behavioural tests which most frequently showed an effect of exposure were those relating to detection of the field or to activity. Most other behavioural tests did not change with electric-field exposure at field strengths up to 100 kV/m. Table 2 includes a summary of experimental results from nervous system and behavioural studies in animals.

5.4 Sensory Phenomena

Strong electric fields cause hairs to oscillate. The movement of hairs on the ear tips of swine was detected photographically in 60-Hz electric fields at 50 kV/m (Kaune et al., 1980); rat vibrissae movement was observed in a 50 Hz, 50 kV/m field by Cabanes & Gary (1981). Stern et al. (1983) attempted to examine field sensitivity thresholds in nude or shaved rats, but saw little difference from results with fur-bearing subjects.

Jaffe (in press) observed a direct field effect on mechanoreceptors of the cat paw above a threshold local electric field strength of 220 kV/m.

Extraordinarily sensitive electroreceptive capabilities exist in some species (e.g., Elasmobranch fish), particularly where there has been evolutionary adaptation to refine sensory organs (Kalmijn, 1966; Bullock, 1973).

Cues, including magnetic field direction, seem important in birds (Walcott, 1974) and in several species ranging from bacteria and bees (where ferromagnetic materials have been found) (Gould et al., 1978) to dolphins and man (Blakemore et al., 1979), although the data in man are disputed. These findings highlight the fact that extrapolation of the results of experimental amimal studies to man is quite complex. Allowances must be made for differences in species sensitivities to ELF fields.

5.5 Effects on the Haematopoietic System in Animals

Numerous studies on animals (Bianchi et al., 1973; Cerretelli & Malaguti, 1976; LeBars & Andre, 1976; Graves, 1977; Graves et al., 1979; Marino & Becker, 1977; Cerretelli et al., 1979; Phillips et al., 1979; Conti et al., 1981; Ragan et al., 1983) concern field-related variations in blood cell populations. There is evidence in these studies of a prompt effect on neutrophilic cells and possibly an effect on thrombocytes and reticulocytes. The data do not permit determination of possible mechanisms that may involve either an effect of the internal fields directly on haematopoietic tissues, or an effect on tissues affected via the central

Table 2. Nervous system and behavioural studies in animals

Exposure (kV/m)	Frequency (Hz)	Subject	Effects examined	Reference
0.0074	60	monkey	no effect on operant behaviour	deLorge (1973)
up to 0.056	45, 60, 75	monkey	altered behaviour (frequency specific)	Gavalas-Medici & Day-Magdaleno (1976)
0.01 - 0.056	7, 10	monkey	changes in interresponse time, dose-dependent. EEG entrainment at field frequency	Gavalas et al. (1970)
0.1	60	rat	no effect in preference behaviour or in temporal discrimination	deLorge & Marr (1974)
up to 0.1	45	mouse	no effect on brain and serum serotonin	Krueger & Reed (1975)
up to 0.1	45	rat	altered brain acetyl transferase	Noval et al. (1976)
0.8 - 1.2	60	mouse	more active in dark periods	Moos (1964)
4.2	60	bees	increased activity during exposure	Greenberg & Bindokas (1981)
up to 25	60	rat	initial startle reaction	Stern et al. (1980)
2 - 10	60	rat	detection threshold approximately 8 kV/m	Stern et al. (1983)
25,50	60	mouse	initial sterile reaction	Graves (1977)
25, 50	60	rat	preference for area of exposure	Hjeresen et al. (1980)
26	60	chick	peck suppression, 28% decrease in motor activity	Graves et al. (1978)
30	60	swine	perception of field, prefer shielded area at night	Hjeresen et al. (1982)

30	60	rat	no effect in taste aversion	Creim et al. (1980)
30	60	baboon	small behavioural changes	Feldstone et al. (1980)
32	60	pigeon	perception of field altered in exposed animals	Graves et al. (1978)
10 - 75	60	mouse	transient hyperactivity in inactive phase, 35 kV/m average threshold	Ehret et al. (1980b) Rosenberg et al. (1983)
40	60	chicks	decreased activity in exposed animals	Bankoske et al. (1976) Graves et al. (1978)
50	50	mouse, rat, guinea-pig	no effect on behaviour	Le Bars et al. (1983)
10 - 75	60	mouse	hyperactivity with intermittent exposure (commencing at 50 kV/m)	Rosenberg et al. (1983)
67	60	chicken	no effect on activity or gross behaviour	Bankoske et al. (1976)
67	60	mouse	hyperactivity with intermittent exposure	Ehret et al. (1980a,b)
75, 90, 100	60	rat	rats spend more time out of field	Hjeresen et al. (1980)
80	60	cat	EEG changes	Silney (1979)
65[a]	60	rat	increased excitability of sympathetic ganglion	Jaffe et al. (1980)
65[a]	60	rat	no effect on peripheral nerve function	Jaffe et al. (1980
65[a]	60	rat	excitatory changes in neuromuscular function; slower recovery from fatigue	Jaffe et al. (1981)
100	60	rat	aversion behaviour	Lovely (1982)

[a] Effective field strength.

nervous system as a result of peripheral sensory stimuli. In all cases, the changes in peripheral leukocyte counts have been within the range of physiological norms. A summary of studies on the haematopoietic system in animals is presented in Table 3.

5.6 Cardiovascular Effects

Cardiovascular function can be assessed by measuring blood pressure and heart rate and by performing ECGs. So far, reported evidence of changes in cardiovascular function has been limited and contradictory. In early studies, a decrease was reported in the heart rate and cardiac output of dogs exposed to 15 kV/m (Gann, 1976), and an increase in heart rate in chickens exposed to 80 kV/m (Carter & Graves, 1975). Comprehensive studies in rats showed no effects from exposure to 100 kV/m (Hilton & Phillips, 1980). Transient increases in blood pressure in dogs exposed to field strengths greater than 10 kV/m have been reported (Cerretelli & Malaguti, 1976).

5.7 Effects on Endocrinology and Blood Chemistry

A large body of data has been collected under different exposure conditions on measurements of different blood plasma proteins, enzymes, etc. Some of these data are summarized in Table 4. No consistent picture of physiological or pathological changes is evident.

Many of the major hormones have been examined for the effects of electric-field exposure, particularly in rats and mice (Phillips et al., 1979). Possible effects have been observed in only three: corticosterone, testosterone, and melatonin. Because corticosterone is produced by the body in response to stress, blood levels of the hormone are extremely sensitive to the method used in obtaining samples. Perhaps because of this sensitivity (rather than the effects of electric-field exposure), a number of laboratories have reported conflicting results.

5.8 Effects on the Immune System

In considering the pattern of effects on white cell populations, it is of special importance to evaluate the immunocompetence of electric-field-exposed animals. Schneider & Kaune (1981) did not find any effects on the response to infection in chicks exposed to 2 kV/m. Morris & Phillips (1982, 1983) did not find any effects on cell-mediated or humoral immune response in rats or mice exposed to fields of 0.2 kV/m. No effect was observed from electric-field exposure on infectivity by a leukemogenic virus in chickens (Phillips

Table 3. Haematopoietic studies in animals

Exposure (kV/m)	Frequency (Hz)	Subject	Effects	Reference
0.01	50	mouse	altered leukocyte distribution	Blanchi et al. (1973)
0.01	50	rat	altered leukocyte distribution	Blanchi et al. (1973)
0.01	45, 60	rat	all effects within normal range	Mathewson et al. (1977)
5	60	mouse	decrease in RBC concentrations	Marino & Becker (1977)
10	50	dog	no effect on haematology	Cerretelli et al. (1979)
10	50	dog	no effect on haematology	Conti et al. (1981)
25	60	mouse	higher WBC count	Graves et al. (1979)
25	50	dog	altered leukocyte distribution, RBC count and haemoglobin	Cerretelli & Malaguti (1976)
50	50	rabbit	altered total leukocytes and RBC	LeBars & Andre (1976)
50	50	rat	no effect on haematology	LeBars & Andre (1976)
50	50	rat, mouse, guinea-pig	no effect on haematology	LeBars et al. (1983)
50	60	mouse	higher WBC count	Graves et al. (1979)

Table 3 (contd).

Exposure (kV/m)	Frequency (Hz)	Subject	Effects	Reference
65	60	rat	increased leukocytes in *in utero*-exposed offspring	Phillips et al. (1979)
65	60	rat	no effect on haematology	Ragan et al. (1983)
65	60	mouse	WBC increased in F_2 generation females	Phillips et al. (1979)
65	60	mouse	RBC increased in F_2 generation offspring	Phillips et al. (1979)
90	60	rat	no effect on polychromatic RBCs	Phillips et al. (1979)
100	50	rat	altered leukocyte distribution	Cerretelli & Malaguti (1976)
100	50	rat	significant changes in blood morphology and chemistry	Cerretelli et al. (1979)
100[a]	60	rat	no effect on haematology	Ragan et al. (1983)
100	50	rat	significant changes in blood morphology and chemistry	Conti et al. (1981)
100	60	rat	increased leukocytes in *in utero*-exposed animals	Phillips et al. (1979)
100	60	rat	no effect on haematology or serum chemistry	Ragan et al. (1983)

[a] 65 kV/m effective.

Table 4. Studies on endocrinology and blood chemistry

Exposure (kV/m)	Frequency (Hz)	Subject	Effects	Reference
0.1	45	rat	altered plasma corticosterone levels	Noval et al. (1976)
0.1	45	rat	no effects on serum chemistry	Mathewson et al. (1977)
1.5	60	rat	lower melatonin in pineal gland	Wilson et al. (1981, 1983)
5	60	rat	no effects on serum chemistry	Marino & Becker (1977)
10	60	rat	adrenal response elevated	Lymangrover et al. (1983)
15	60	rat	lower serum corticosterone	Marino et al. (1976a)
15	60	rat	lower albumin	Marino & Becker (1977)
15	60	dog	no effects on cortisol secretion	Gann (1976)
25	50	dog	no effects	Cerretelli & Malaguti (1976)
25, 50	60	mouse	transient effect on steroid concentrations	Graves (1977)

Table 4 (contd).

Exposure (kV/m)	Frequency (Hz)	Subject	Effects	Reference
50	50	rabbit	altered calcium, glucose, urea	LeBars & Andre (1976)
50	50	mouse	no effects on blood biochemistry	LeBars et al. (1983)
50	50	rat	no effects	LeBars & Andre (1976); LeBars et al. (1983)
50	50	guinea-pig	no effects on blood biochemistry	LeBars et al. (1983)
65	60	rat	lower testosterone levels (120-day exposures); no effects in other hormones	Free et al. (1981)
80	60	rat	no change in corticosterone level	Seto et al. (1982)
100[a]	60	rat	no effects on serum chemistry	Ragan et al. (1983)
100	50	rat	no effects	Cerretelli & Malaguti (1976)

[a] 65 kV/m effective.

et al., 1981). Lyle et al. (1983), however, observed significant decrements in the cytolytic capacity of lymphocytes exposed to radiofrequency fields modulated at 60 Hz. In an extensive study, Le Bars et al. (1983) found no significant effects on immune response of rats, mice, or guinea-pigs exposed to 50 kV/m, 50 Hz electric fields for 8, 14, or 18 h/day over periods varying from 1 to 6 months.

Evidence from many blood studies on man or laboratory animals shows slight changes in white cell populations, almost always within the range of normal values. These shifts may, however, indicate some alterations involving the immune system. Further research is indicated, before a conclusion can be reached. Overall, the evidence from many studies indicates that animal morbidity and mortality in long-term exposures is unaffected, suggesting that the immune response is generally unaffected.

5.9 Growth and Development Studies

Data from many studies on rats, mice, or chickens (Knickerbocker et al., 1967; Marino et al., 1974; Krueger et al., 1975; Bankoske et al., 1976; Cerretelli & Malaguti, 1976; LeBars & Andre, 1976; Noval et al., 1976; Mathewson et al., 1977; Cerretelli et al., 1979; Graves et al., 1979; Phillips et al., 1979, 1981; Fam, 1980; Conti et al., 1981; Greenberg & Bindokas, 1981; Le Bars et al., 1983; Portet, 1983) suggest that there are no effects on growth and development. In particular, the data from multi-generation studies on mice do not indicate any pattern of an effect on these parameters.

Exceptions are reported in two instances. Severe stunting was reported in a wild strain of rabbits reared outdoors in a substation electric field of 14 kV/m (50 Hz) in comparison with rabbits in an electric field-free cage (Hansson, 1981a,b). The same author did not find any growth changes in rabbits exposed under indoor laboratory conditions. Secondly, the results of multi-generation studies in electric-field-exposed swine (30 kV/m) and rats (65 kV/m) revealed developmental defects that included an increased incidence of fetal malformations in two successive generations of miniature swine exposed for 18 months and in one of two rat generations (Phillips, 1981, 1983; Sikov, 1982; Anderson & Phillips, 1984). Because of the important implications of these studies, additional research should be conducted to address questions that, at present, preclude conclusions concerning a cause and effect relationship between the various fields used in these studies and the observed effects on development. In particular, in the swine or rat studies, similar effects were not seen in all generations, and the influence of environmental stress in the rabbit study requires clarification. A summary of some of the results of growth and development studies is given in Table 5.

5.10 Reproduction and Fertility

Studies on reproductive function have been carried out at many field strengths (Knickerbocker et al., 1967; Krueger et al., 1975; Phillips et al., 1979; Sikov et al., 1979) with no evidence of consistent electric-field effects in rats or mice.

Effects on rat, swine, rabbit, and chicken growth and development are described in the previous section. Swine conceived, born, and then kept in the electric field for 18 months showed a deficit in mating performance (Phillips, 1981). A summary of effects on fertility and reproduction is presented in Table 6.

5.11 Mutagenesis

Results of studies on Drosophila (Mittler, 1972; Bender, 1976) did not indicate any mutagenic effects, though those of an earlier study (Coate & Negerbon, 1970) had suggested effects. Other studies (Knickerbocker et al., 1967; Krueger et al., 1975) did not show any effects.

No effects have been observed that would suggest that electric-field exposure is mutagenic (Phillips et al., 1979; Frazier et al., 1982).

5.12 Circadian Rhythms in Animals

Apart from the extensive investigations of Wever (1968) on alterations in circadian rhythms in human beings, only a few studies have been conducted to examine the effects of electric fields on natural biological rhythms. Ehret et al. (1980a,b) measured rat metabolism but did not observe any effects on the circadian rhythms of metabolism in animals exposed to 8.2 kV/m, or on ultradian rhythm in fields up to 100 kV/m. Wilson et al. (1981, 1983) examined circadian rhythms in rats in a more direct fashion, measuring the cyclical pineal production of indolamines and enzymes. A significant reduction in the normal night-time rise of melatonin and biosynthetic enzymes was observed in rats exposed to either 1.5 or 40 kV/m. Furthermore, the change in pineal indole response occurred only after 3 weeks of chronic exposure (Anderson et al., 1982).

5.13 Bone Growth and Repair

McClanahan & Phillips (1983) reported that bone growth in rats did not appear to be affected by exposure to 100 kV/m. Marino et al. (1979) and McClanahan & Phillips (1983) reported

Table 5. Studies on growth and development

Exposure (kV/m or mT)	Frequency (Hz)	Subject	Effect	Reference
0.1	45	rat	no effect on body weight	Mathewson et al. (1977)
0.1	45	rat	altered growth	Noval et al. (1976)
3.4	45 or 75	chick	no effect on body weight	Krueger & Reed (1975)
3.5 (0.1 - 3 mT)	45, 60, or 75	chick	no effect on posthatching growth and development	Durfee et al. (1975)
5 and 15	60	rat	decreased body weight	Marino et al. (1976, 1980)
7	60	bee	no effect on bee or hive weight	Greenberg et al. (1979)
10 and 15	60	mouse	decreased body weight	Marino et al. (1976)
14	50	rabbit	stunted growth (raised outdoors)	Hansson (1981a,b)
15	60	rat	increased pituitary and adrenal weights in exposed	Marino et al. (1976)
25	60	mouse	no effect on development	Phillips et al. (1981)
25	50	rat	lower growth rate	Cerretelli et al. (1979); Conti et al. (1981)
30	60	swine	no effect on body weight	Phillips et al. (1979)
30	60	swine	increased rate of fetal malformations (in 2 generations)	Phillips et al. (1981); Phillips (1983)

Table 5 (contd).

Exposure (kV/m)	Frequency (Hz)	Subject	Effect	Reference
50	50	rabbit	no effect on growth	LeBars & Andre (1976)
50	50	mouse, rat, guinea-pig	no effect on growth	LeBars et al. (1983)
50	50	rat	no effect on growth	Portet (1983)
65	60	rat	increased rate of fetal malformations (1 of 2 generations)	Phillips (1983)
67	50	chicken	no effect on body weight	Bankoske et al. (1976)
80	60	chick	no effect on body weight	Graves et al. (1979)
80	50	chick	no effect on growth	Bankoske et al. (1976)
100	50	rat	no effect on embryo morphology	Cerretelli & Malaguti (1976)
100	50	rat	lower growth rate	Cerretellí et al. (1979); Conti et al. (1981)
100	60	rat	no effect on growth	Phillips et al. (1979)
160	60	mouse	lower body weight in offspring of exposed males	Knickerbocker et al. (1967)

Table 6. Studies on fertility and reproduction

Exposure (kV/m)	Frequency (Hz)	Subject	Effect	Reference
1.6 (or 1.2 G)	60	chicken	reduced egg production	Krueger et al. (1975)
3.4	60	chicken	no effects on hatchability, embryonic morphology, or sex ratios	Krueger et al. (1975)
3.5 (or 1 - 3 G)	45, 60, or 75	chicken	no effects on hatchability, embryonic survival	Durfee et al. (1975)
10 or 15	60	mouse	no effects on litters or litter size	Marino et al. (1976)
30	60	swine (F_0)	no effects on farrowing success rate (1st breeding)	Phillips (1981)
30	60	swine (F_0)	increase in fetal abnormalities (2nd breeding)	Phillips (1981)
30	60	swine (F_1)	poor breeding performance	Phillips (1981)
30	60	swine (F_1)	increased fetal abnormalities (1st breeding)	Phillips (1983)

Table 6 (contd).

Exposure (kV/m)	Frequency (Hz)	Subject	Effect	Reference
50	50	rat	no effect on estrus cycle	LeBars & Andre (1976)
67	60	chickens	no effects on hatchability or time to hatch	Bankoske et al. (1976)
100	50	rat	effect on numbers of matings and pregnancies	Cerretelli & Malaguti (1976)
100	50	rat	no effect on fertility	Cerretelli et al. (1979); Conti et al. (1981)
100	60	mouse	no effects on fertility, mortality, size of litter, sex ratio	Phillips et al. (1979)
100	60	rat	no effects on mortality, litter size, or reproductive performance	Sikov et al. (1979)
100	60	rat	earlier development of motor activity	Phillips et al. (1979)
160	60	mouse	no effect on reproductive ability	Knickerbock et al. (1967)

that bone-fracture repair was retarded in rats and mice exposed to fields as low as 5 kV/m but not in animals exposed to very low (1 kV/m) field strengths. Exposure may affect the rate of healing but not the strength of the healed bone (McClanahan & Phillips, 1983).

5.14 The Problems of Extrapolating Animal Exposure Data to Human Beings

Because either the surface electric field or the internal current density at a particular organ varies with the size, shape, and orientation of the body, no single animal model can successfully simulate the exposure conditions of a human being. At best, a single study can approximate human exposures either to the surface fields at a selected spot, or to the internal current density in a selected organ (Sheppard & Eisenbud, 1977; Kaune & Phillips, 1980).

Kaune & Phillips (1980) calculated the current through various sections of the body, and from the cross-sectional area, calculated the average current density for the rat, swine, or human being exposed to the same (unperturbed) electric field. The data showed very large differences in currents as a function of animal posture. For example, the total neck current in a horizontal rat exposed to a 10-kV/m vertical E field was 1.6 μA, but, when the rat reared, the current increased to 3.2 μA. The respective current densities were 28 and 140 nA/cm². An even larger ratio of about 7-fold occurred for the chest currents, while, in the abdomen, the resting rat had a current density of only 2 nA/cm² compared with 85 nA/cm² in the rearing rat. In either case, because of the larger capacitance of the human body, the current density in the human neck will be greater than that in the rat.

According to the foregoing considerations, for example, a study designed to examine the effects of electric current density in the neck of a man exposed to 10 kV/m would, if conducted on rats, require an electric field of 200 kV/m, or in the case of pigs, 140 kV/m, whereas studies involving animals that stand erect more often (such as primates) would require lower field strengths (Kaune & Phillips, 1980). An electric field that produced a reasonable match between man and the test animal in one part of the body would tend to overexpose other parts of the animal body, for example, the limbs.

Another approach to the determination of relative exposures between man and animals considers the "enhancement factors" for the surface electric field. Deno (1977) reported that, for human beings, the surface electric field at the top of the head was 18 times that of the unperturbed electric field, whereas at the back of the head the enhancement was 15 fold. At the upper arm, an 8-fold enhancement occurred for the size and shape parameters given by Deno. When a rat was exposed to a 10-kV/m unperturbed electric field, the maximum field strength of 37 kV/m occurred at the back, while an upright man in the same field had a maximum field of 180 kV/m at the top of the head (Kaune & Phillips, 1980).

These data indicate that man's size and posture make it difficult to simulate in laboratory animals the current densities that occur when man is exposed to strong electric fields. Because of the interference of artifactual shocks, hair stimulation, corona, and other problems of extremely high voltage, it is not practical to expose animals to levels much higher than 100 kV/m.

The species differences between man and laboratory animals may strongly affect the threshold for biological response, the magnitude of a physiological response, and the degree of adaption. Biochemical differences among species may also prove significant. None of these species-dependency factors is understood in the context of ELF electric field exposures.

Magnetic field exposures may require scaling according to body size, shape, and orientation if the primary action is due to the induced electric field. The magnetic field itself is not perturbed by either animal or human bodies and is essentially unchanged at points outside or inside the body.

6. HUMAN STUDIES

6.1 Sources of Information

Three sources of information exist concerning the effects on man of exposure to ELF fields:

(a) surveys of the state of health of high-voltage linemen, utility, substation, and switch-yard workers;

(b) epidemiological studies of inhabitants near high-voltage transmission lines, power distribution lines, and substations; and

(c) examination of volunteers exposed to ELF fields under controlled conditions.

Additional information can be obtained from follow-up studies of patients exposed to ELF fields as a result of medical applications. Except for a report by Bassett (1981) on the state of patient health, information is related to the effectiveness of the applied medical procedure.

Although there is no good substitute for reliable epidemiological data for the evaluation of general population and occupational health aspects of ELF exposure, data from present studies are insufficient to draw any firm conclusions. However, other epidemiological studies are in progress which may provide further information needed to establish better health criteria (Baroncelli et al., 1984; Checcucci, 1984; Knave, 1984).

6.2 Study Design

In epidemiological studies, it is difficult to obtain quantitative, unbiased data that can be reliably interpreted. Two problems with most of the human studies to date are the failure to obtain measurement data on the level and duration of exposure, and the failure to include an appropriate control group that is comparable in all respects to the exposed group, except for exposure to the electromagnetic field. While this does not necessarily invalidate the results of such studies, these shortcomings must be taken into account.

End-points can be selected to ascertain the health impact of ELF exposure in areas of particular public concern. Effects on the nervous system, behaviour, the cardiovascular system, tumour incidence, reproductive success, or development are among the appropriate end-points. Some authors (Utidjian, 1979) maintain that, because there is no basis for postulating a specific disease or cause of death related to ELF exposure, epidemiological studies need to be cross-sectional, evaluating the general state of health and the incidence of diseases. A basic problem is the selection of appropriate matched control groups. Other, often overlooked problems include those of obtaining appropriate information on exposure duration and levels, the occurrence of confounding factors, as well as the need for differentiation between the effects of ELF exposure and the influence of collateral phenomena such as noise, microshocks, ozone, or possibly the presence of various ions and chemical substances.

Finally, to prevent the introduction of bias, all studies should be "blind". This means that, whenever possible, personnel who record data should be unaware of the subjects' exposure history.

6.3 Health Status of Occupationally-Exposed Human Beings

A summary of studies on the health status of linemen and switch-yard workers is given in Table 7.

Asanova & Rakov (1966) examined 45 high-voltage switch-yard workers. This survey indicated a variety of symptoms in the cardiovascular, digestive, and central nervous systems subsequent to prolonged exposure of switch-yard workers to electric fields (up to 26 kV/m). The disturbances noted were subjective. No control group was examined. Furthermore, recent work in the USSR has suggested that the observed effects might be the result of exposure to microshocks or kerosene vapour rather than to electric fields (Danilin et al., 1969; Savin et al., 1978; Bourgsdorf, 1980).

Results from the earliest comparable studies in the USA failed to confirm those of the USSR studies. Kouwenhoven et al. (1967) and Singewald et al. (1973) who studied 10 linemen exposed during their work (4-year period) to unperturbed fields of up to 25 kV/m did not observe any correlation between exposure and the health of the subjects. However, this study included only a small number of subjects, and descriptions of the experimental protocol and results were incomplete.

Sazonova (1967) reported on physiological tests performed on 400 - 500 kV substation workers divided into 2 groups according to the presumed extent of electric field exposure. The high electric-field-exposed group had significantly lower blood pressure, greater neuromuscular activity, and increased latent reaction times and higher error rates in a stimulus-response test. The exposure information was not adequate to determine either electric field strength or duration of exposure.

Table 7. Studies on the health status of linemen and switch-yard workers

Reference	No. of subjects	Comments
Kouwenhoven et al. (1967); Singewald et al. (1973)	10	Linemen, 10-year period of observation, only general medical data, no effects reported, no data on exposure levels, no control groups; same subjects in both studies
Asanova & Rakov (1966)	45	Switch-yard workers (500 kV): subjective and objective indications of functional neurovegetative disturbances; exposure estimated; no control group; Danilin et al. (1969) suggested that chemical pollution (kerosene) may have been responsible
Sazonova (1967)	211	Switch-yard workers (400 - 500 kV): exposure estimated; neurovegetative disturbances (as above); increased latent reaction time and error rates; no control group
Revnova et al. (1968)	114	Switch-yard workers (500 kV): findings as Asanova & Rakov (1966); inadequate data on exposure; no control group
Danilin et al. (1969)	12	Switch-yard workers: detailed clinical (hospitalization) study; average exposure 14 kV/m, maximum 26 kV/m; no effects; no control group

Table 7 (contd).

Reference	No. of subjects	Comments
Fole et al. (1974); Fole (1973)	9	Switch-yard workers transferred from a 200 kV to a 400 kV substation: exposures up to 15 kV/m; findings as Asanova & Rakov (1966) plus visual troubles; no control group
Malboysson (1976)	160	84 switch-yard workers and 76 HV-linemen compared to 94 controls (low-voltage linemen): questionnaires and medical examinations; no effects, better health of HV-workers; inadequate data on exposure; no statistical analysis
Roberge (1976)	160	Switch-yard workers (735 kV): inadequate data on exposure; no health effects; electric shock anxiety; ratio male/female offspring 17:3; no control group
Stopps & Janischensky (1979)	30	Linemen compared to 30 matched controls from among the power company employees: clinical studies, including ECG and EEG; no effects; exposed group was preselected (volunteers); exposures extrapolated from measurements
Knave et al. (1979)	53	400 kV station workers matched with 53 unexposed power company employees: no differences in health status; comprehensive medical and psychological study; good exposure data
Issel et al. (1977)	110	Linemen working on 110 and 380 kV lines with protective clothing; no effects; control group used
Broadbent et al. (in press)	390	Questionnaires on linemen and switch-yard workers; 28 exposed above level of detection threshold of monitor; control group; no effects found

Revnova et al. (1968) carried out a study on 114 workers (99 males, 15 females) in a 500 kV substation with findings similar to those of Asanova & Rakov (1966). Danilin et al. (1969) did not report any adverse health effects in a clinical study on 12 workers exposed to an average field strength of 14 kV/m, which generated whole body currents of 130 μA (maximum 26 kV/m and 230 μA). Krivova et al. (1973) found no physiological changes at 10 kV/m, but did identify some impairment of motor skills after exposure for 2 h to 16 kV/m.

To assess the health status of electricians on high voltage systems, an investigation was started in the German Democratic Republic in 1971 (Kupfer & Issel, 1975). The subjects included linemen wearing protective clothing who worked bare-handed on 110 - 380 kV lines (Jahn et al., 1978). The men were examined according to clinical criteria (locomotion system, cardiovascular system, respiration system, haematopoietic system, kidney and liver function, eyes, ears, and nose) and psychological criteria (risk-taking behaviour, motivation, sensomotor coordination, reaction time, intellectual abilities for technical thinking, personality). Examination of 110 linemen and fitters did not reveal any health changes or injuries attributable to the 50-Hz fields (Issel et al., 1977). Electric fitters exposed under similar physiological and psychological conditions, but at a field strength of 5 kV/m, served as a control group.

In Spain, Fole (1973) and Fole et al. (1974) reported subjective health effects among 6 workers from a 400-kV substation; there was no control group. A group of 84 substation workers and 76 linemen in Spain were compared with 94 linemen working on low voltage systems (Malboysson, 1976). The linemen in both groups showed no apparent adverse effects due to work in electric fields. No exposure measurements were taken, and the data were not statistically analysed.

Knave et al. (1979) examined 53 workers at 400 kV-substations in comparison with a matched reference group of 53 unexposed workers. Only occasional exposures to field strengths above 5 kV/m occurred (Table 8). Data on subjective complaints were collected using standard questionnaires and interviews. Eight psychological tests were performed. EEGs and ECGs were recorded, blood pressure measured, and peripheral blood cell counts were made. No biochemical tests were made. Comparison of substation workers and the reference group generally showed no observation of a lower number of offspring. However, a lower rate of male offspring was observed but not attributed to electric field exposure.

In an earlier study (Roberge, 1976), 56 switch-yard workers at 735-kV substations in Quebec, Canada were examined. A questionnaire oriented towards nervous system complaints was used, and a clinical examination that included

Table 8. Percentage (%) of working time spent in electric fields of different strengths by 400-kV substation workers[a]

Type of work	E-field strength ranges (kV/m)			
	0 - 5	5 - 10	10 - 15	15 - 20
Inspection rounds	66	37	2	1
Everyday work	34	61	4.8	0.2
Breaker work:				
Revision	60	0	18	16
Testing	95	5	0	0

[a] From: Knave et al. (1979).

an ECG and a thorough examination of the peripheral blood chemistry, was conducted. The data were compared with "normal" reference values rather than those of a control group. Differences in eosinophil number (P < 0.05) were, however, within clinical norms, and of doubtful statistical value.

Stopps & Janischewsky (1979) studied 30 high-voltage maintenance men and 30 matched employees not exposed to electric fields. Clinical and psychological investigations were made in a hospital. In the exposed group, 19 linemen had estimated exposures of 7 kV/m h per day (up to 8000 kV/m h over 10 years); and 11 substation workers had average estimated exposures of 13 kV/m h per day (up to 36 000 kV/m h over 10 years). No adverse health effects were found.

A health-questionnaire study (Broadbent et al., in press) was conducted on 390 electrical power transmission and distribution workers employed in the electrical industry in the United Kingdom, of whom 28 were exposed to levels above the detection threshold of the dosemeter. Actual exposure levels, measured during the two weeks prior to the questionnaire interview, were considerably less that the estimated exposures. About 150 interview questions were administered by industrial nurses. Each man was asked to assess his own experience of headaches in the last 6 months on a scale 0 - 3. Visits to doctors over six months and taking of prescribed or unprescribed medicines were noted. A measure of cognitive failure, i.e., frequency of minor episodes of forgetfulness or inattention, was measured. Although there were significant differences in the health effect measurements between different job categories and different parts of the country, no significant correlation was found between these effects and exposures to electric fields.

Five preliminary observations were reported, four published as "letters to the editor", of an increase in the incidence of leukaemia in groups of workers loosely defined as "electrical workers" (Milham, 1982; Wright et al., 1982; Coleman et al., 1983; McDowall, 1983; Vagero & Olin, 1983).

Milham (1982) reported on a data base of 438 000 deaths of men, who were 20 years of age or older and were residents of Washington State, USA, from 1950-79. A proportional mortality ratio (PMR = observed/expected x 100) due to leukaemia, significant at the $\underline{P} < 0.01$ level, was observed for "electricians", TV and radio repairmen, power station operators, and aluminium workers. Wright et al. (1982) sought to verify Milham's (1982) results by examining a similar statistic, the proportional incidence ratio (PIR) of a different and much smaller data base. They found significant increases ($\underline{P} < 0.05$) in the incidence of acute myeloid leukaemia (on the basis of a total of 4 cases) in power linemen and telephone linemen, two groups for which the Washington data yielded insignificant PMRs.

Additional data on occupational leukaemia rates in the United Kingdom were provided in two letters. McDowall (1983) found an increased evidence of leukaemia in occupationally-exposed electrical workers using PMRs and also by a case-control study. Coleman et al. (1983) also examined the leukaemia incidence for the same electrical occupations with evidence of a 17% excess that was especially strong for electrical fitters and telegraph operators, for whom the extent of electric or magnetic field exposure was not established.

These occupational groups have a number of environmental factors in common, viz, exposure to electromagnetic fields and a variety of metals and chemical fluxes. Electricians working in homes usually work on equipment that is not operating or operates at low voltages. Telecommunication and electronic personnel are normally exposed to levels of power frequency electric or magnetic fields no higher than those encountered in the average modern home. These reports are inadequate in many ways for use in determining if there is any association between leukaemia and exposure to electric or magnetic fields. However, they merit further detailed study to elucidate the signficance of the findings.

Finally, Vagero & Olin (1983) examined data from the Swedish Cancer Environment Registry for the incidence of all types of cancer among electrical or electronic industry workers compared with the general working population. The authors claimed a nearly two-fold excess of pharyngeal cancers among the test population. However, the accuracy of the job classifications over the relevant time periods was questionable. The authors were careful to point out that caution was needed for any conclusions with regard to relationships.

The association of electrical occupation with leukaemia suggested in these studies was not consistent and often involved very few disease cases in an occupational category. Deficiencies in these studies could be summarized as follows (Repacholi, 1984a):

(a) lack of consistency in designating occupational classification;

(b) no account was taken of mobility between occupations; and

(c) occupational groups sharing exposure to electric and magnetic fields were undoubtedly exposed to other physical and chemical agents.

In studies such as these, associations can be detected with a reasonable degree of certainty, if appropriate statistics are applied to a large enough data base of good integrity. The suggestion of field-related leukaemia raises important questions that should be addressed using studies of adequate statistical power in which exposure is more accurately determined.

Bauchinger et al. (1981) examined the chromosomes in blood lymphocytes of 32 switch-yard workers (380 kV) and did not find any differences in comparison with matched, unexposed workers. However, the control group demonstrated a rather high incidence of chromatid gaps, 17 ± 1.3 per 1000 cells, compared with the "positive" control group of nuclear power plant workers (15.0 ± 1.0 per 1000 cells). In Sweden (Nordström et al., 1981), preliminary work has been described in which increased frequency of chromosome breakage was seen in a few workers exposed to 400 kV. Furthermore, congenital deformities were found in 10% of 119 children of substation workers, whereas only 2.7% of children of unexposed workers showed such deformities (Nordström et al., 1983). Analyses of these data raise major questions in the interpretation of the results, because the highest percentage of abnormal progeny appears to be related to type of job rather than to level of exposure (Anderson & Phillips, 1984).

More research is this area is necessary in properly-designed human studies of significant magnitude to establish whether any asociation exists between exposure to ELF and induction of chromosome aberrations.

Nordström & Birke (1979) carried out a retrospective study on the incidence of congenital malformation in the progeny of 542 male employees of the Swedish State Power Board. The increased frequency of malformations reported in this study occurred evenly throughout the populations studied, irrespective of whether they worked in 400 kV, 130 - 200 kV, or 70 kV situations.

Employees exposed to very low level ELF electric fields (generally less than 0.05 V/m and accompanying magnetic flux of densities 10^{-5} T) at the site of a test communications antenna (Project Sanquine) did not show any pathological effects related to the fields. In particular, an investigation for neurological symptoms did not reveal any effects (Krumpe & Tockman, 1974).

6.4 Studies on the General Population

Wertheimer & Leeper (1979) reported a two- to three-fold increase in the incidence of leukaemia among Colorado children presumably exposed to magnetic fields of strengths up to 0.7 μT. Magnetic fields were estimated by scoring the type of electrical wiring configuration close to the homes (power lines of various voltages and current-carrying capacity) into categories of high- or low-current configurations.

The same authors (Wertheimer & Leeper, 1982), extended their work to a study of the incidence of adult cancer in people living near high-current electric wiring. The associations suggested were not dependent on age, urbanism, neighbourhood, or socio-economic level and were more clearly demonstrated when urban/industrial factors were not present to obscure the pattern. The four types of cancer that appeared to be particularly elevated in the exposed adult populations were cancer of the nervous system, uterus, breast, and lymphomas. The authors suggested that magnetic fields might have a promoter effect since the increases were maximal, 7 years from the time of taking up residence in the area.

These preliminary studies have limitations common to many epidemiological studies involving cohort selection. Additional problems include possible biases in the techniques for scoring the wiring configurations, and in the assumption that the scoring does accurately segregate magnetic field strength levels among the cases examined.

Further questions are raised since the data were not collected blind and cases were ascertained after death, no account being taken of cancer cases still alive. Furthermore, both birth and death addresses were used, which introduces a potential for observer bias.

Considerable interest has been provoked by these findings and it is expected that many of the issues will be dealt with in follow-up studies.

The hypothesis that such weak magnetic fields (of the order of 0.1 - 0.7 μT) induce biological effects has raised questions such as those of Miller (1980), who criticized the Wertheimer & Leeper studies on the basis that the magnetic field from electrical appliances in the home would far exceed any contributions from electrical wiring configurations in the environment.

A similar study carried out by Fulton et al. (1980) in Rhode Island failed to reveal any evidence to support the Wertheimer and Leeper hypothesis. However, Wertheimer & Leeper (1980) reanalysed the Rhode Island data using their own study method and found a slight association of childhood cancer with electrical wiring configuration.

Tomenius et al. (1982) reported a similar finding of increased leukaemia incidence in children living in homes where the levels of the magnetic field measured outside the front door were 0.3 μT or above. The data involved a small number of cases and, again, the field measurement was questionable because the relation of actual exposure to the field outside the home was not established. These studies and the preliminary occupational data (see above) relating some concern to electric or magnetic field exposure must be investigated further to determine if the suggested link with cancer induction or promotion can be established.

6.4.1 Studies on inhabitants of areas in the vicinity of HV-lines

A four-year study on 70 men, 65 women, and 132 children living within 25 metres of 200 and 400 kV lines has been reported by Strumza (1970). The control group consisted of 74 men, 64 women, and 120 children living more than 125 metres from the lines. The author failed to discover any differences between the exposed and control groups on the basis of medical records, frequency of visits to family doctors, or expenditure on pharmaceutical prescriptions. Eckert (1977) tried to establish a relationship between the sudden infant death syndrome and ELF fields, but the method and results were questionable.

In a study by Dumansky et al. (1977), no effects were found in farmers exposed to fields of 12 kV/m for 1.5 h/day. Similarly, Busby et al. (1974) did not find any effects in 18 farmers working on farms in the vicinity of a 765 kV line.

Reichmanis et al. (1979) and Perry et al. (1981) have suggested a link between electromagnetic field exposure and suicide. It has been pointed out (Bonnell et al., 1983) that the reports lack any biological hypothesis. Suicide is frequently a symptom of a pre-existing psychotic illness, and it is these diseases that are important in studying suicide. Furthermore, these authors claimed that the conclusions were contradictory and open to serious criticism on the basis of incorrect use of epidemiological data. The calculation of the magnitude of electric fields was also in error by a factor of 10 000 (Bonnell et al., 1983).

6.5 Studies on Human Volunteers

There is only a limited amount of data on human volunteers exposed to electric fields, low-level currents, or spark discharges under laboratory conditions. These data are valuable because of the greater control over extraneous influences compared with occupational exposures and because they involve the human organism. Of course, studies on human beings are limited to physiological and behavioural observations that do not cause harm and the test sessions are usually relatively short.

In considering these studies, it is important to remember that microshocks can be felt in fields of above 3 kV/m (Takagi & Muto, 1971) and therefore can cause unease in subjects. To assess the effects of the ELF field itself, it is necessary to take care to eliminate the influence of microshocks in the experimental design.

In 1974, R. Hauf and co-workers reported studies on more than 100 human volunteers exposed to 50 Hz electric fields (up to 20 kV/m) during laboratory test sessions that involved relatively brief exposures to the field. In the first report (R. Hauf, 1974), no field-related effects were observed on reaction time, blood pressure, pulse rate, electrocardiogram, or electroencephalogram. Changes in some blood cell variables were seen, but these were within the normal physiological range. Each of the 3-h test sessions included 2 exposures for 45 min to fields at 1, 15, or 20 kV/m, and the testing lasted 3 successive days. Detailed descriptions of the studies are available in the reports of R. Hauf (1974) and Rupilius (1976).

Rupilius (1976) conducted a study on man where 3 days exposure to a 20 kV/m electric field at 50 Hz was combined with exposure to a 0.3 mT magnetic field at 50 Hz. Observations for up to 24 h after exposure showed no changes in blood chemistry, including triglyceride levels. Eisemann (1975) did not show any effects on human subjects exposed for a period of 3 h to a conduction current of 200 μA at 50 Hz, by means of electrodes placed on the ankles and under the arms.

No significant behavioural changes were observed in 20 human subjects exposed to an electric field of 20 kV/m (50 Hz) (Johansson et al., 1973). The exposed subjects performed as well as controls in tests of reaction time and in psychological tests, and responses to a questionnaire did not show any significant differences in perceived levels of discomfort between the test and control groups.

The results of several studies performed by Wever (1968) indicated a significant influence of weak ELF electric fields on human circadian rhythms. He found that the complete absence of electric or magnetic fields led to desynchronisation of certain biorhythms, but that synchronisation was restored by an applied 2.5-V/m, 10-Hz, square-wave electric field. These data are difficult to interpret with reference to electric fields at environmental levels. Wever postulated the existence of a physiological detector of weak electric fields but did not associate this finding with the possibility of health effects from imposed ELF fields.

Human volunteers were also exposed to both electrical fields of 20 kV/m and magnetic fields of 5 mT by Sander et al. (1982). Neither field produced any evident influence on the different parameters studied, except some discontinuous variations in certain of them.

Studies on the nervous system and behaviour in man are summarized in Table 9, and studies on the haematopoietic system, in Table 10.

6.6 Summary

Few physiological or psychological effects in human beings have been credibly related to electric field exposure. Such effects, when reported, have often been questionable for the following reasons (Anderson & Phillips, 1984):

(a) monitoring of symptomatology was subjective and was frequently not well-defined;

(b) quantitative evaluation of effects was either not performed or was not clearly described;

(c) control populations were poorly matched with exposed groups or were absent;

(d) electric fields had been confounded by secondary factors (e.g., microshocks);

(e) observation periods were often short;

(f) exposure levels varied widely or were not documented, making it difficult to estimate accurately the magnitude and duration of exposure;

Table 9. Studies on the nervous system and behaviour in man

Exposure	Frequency (Hz)	Effects examined	Reference
1, 15, or 20 kV/m (up to 2 h)	50	altered reaction time within normal range; no effect on EEG	G. Hauf (1974) R. Hauf (1974) R. Hauf (1976)
20 kV/m, 0.3 mT (for 3 h)	50	no effect on reaction time or EEG	Rupilius (1976) R. Hauf (1976)
0.3 mT	50	no effect on reaction time or EEG	Mantell (1975) R. Hauf (1976)
200 μA (for 3 h)	50	no effect on reaction time or EEG	Eisemann (1975)
6 kV/m (2 x 3 min)	50	effect on EEG when field "on"	Waibel (1975)
380 - 400 kV switch-yards	50	no effect on manual dynamometry	Fole et al. (1974)
400 kV switch-yard workers	50	neuromuscular deficits among exposed workers	Sazonova (1967)
400 kV switch-yard workers	50	various clinical diagnoses related to CNS	Asanova & Rakov (1966)

Table 10. Haematopoietic studies in man

Exposure	Frequency (Hz)	Effect	Reference
1, 15, or 20 kV/m (for 3 h)	50	altered total leukocytes, absolute neutrophils and reticulocytes - all within normal range	G. Hauf (1974) R. Hauf (1974) R. Hauf (1976)
0.3 mT (for 3 h)	50	no effects	Mantell (1975) R. Hauf (1976)
20 KV/m, 0.3 mT	50	no effects	Rupilius (1976) R. Hauf (1976)
200 μA[a]	50	no effects	Eisemann (1975) R. Hauf (1976)
5 mT (for 4 h)	50	no effects outside normal range	Sander et al. (1982)
20 kV/m (6.22 h/day) (for 1 week)	50	no effects outside normal range	Sander et al. (1982)

[a] No field, only conduction current via electrodes (approximately equivalent to exposing man in a 12-kV/m field).

(g) numbers of subjects in many of the earlier studies were insufficient to establish the statistical significance of adverse effects.

7. HEALTH RISK EVALUATION

In making an evaluation of the health risks of exposure to ELF electric and magnetic fields, a number of factors must be considered (Repacholi, 1984a). Criteria must be developed to identify which effects are to be considered a hazard for human health. A distinction needs to be made between the concepts of interaction, biological effect, perception, and hazard.

Difficulty in defining the term health hazard occurs because value judgements are involved that may not be based on scientific analysis. Some may consider any field-induced interaction hazardous. Others suggest that the field is hazardous if it is capable of inducing a physiological perturbation in a biological system that is either measurable or at least theoretically possible. Still others note that a stimulus-producing sensation without pain or discomfort is often assumed to be harmless, but modern research has demonstrated that the opposite may be true (Grissett, 1980).

Interactions that lead to measurable biological effects, which remain within the normal range of physiological compensation of the body and do not detract from the physical and mental well-being of human beings, should not be considered hazardous. Interactions that lead to biological effects outside the normal range of compensation of the body may be an actual or potential health hazard (Repacholi, 1983).

When making a health risk evaluation, strict guidelines must be established prior to reviewing the literature on the biological effects of exposure to static and ELF fields. Certain studies (generally *in vitro*) are conducted to identify underlying mechanisms of interaction. Health risk evaluations cannot be made on the basis of *in vitro* experiments alone, because effects found *in vitro* many not necessarily occur *in vivo*. With *in vitro* experimentation, the toxicity of an agent can be determined in increasingly complex steps. For example, effects on solutions of biological molecules might be used as a model system to study a predominant mechanism of action. Uncomplicated systems can assist in the exploration and evaluation of mechanisms and may serve as a useful basis for designing experiments at the cellular level - the next level of biological complexity. By restricting the complexity of the experimental system, there will be less chance of possible subtle effects being masked by gross or dominant effects.

Thus, health agencies can place only limited value on *in vitro* studies and must await the results of similar or related studies conducted *in vivo*. The *in vitro* results may indicate that a cautious or prudent approach should be adopted when setting standards (Repacholi, 1983). This may be reflected in the development of a safety factor which is applied to the lowest level of exposure at which adverse effects are observed. Once the mechanisms of interaction are understood and found to occur in animals, the next step is to determine if it is possible to extrapolate the results to man.

Unfortunately, the state of knowledge of the interacting mechanisms operating when biological systems are exposed to ELF fields is very limited. At present, it is impossible to furnish any theory to predict the effects of exposure to these fields. Because of this lack of information, care must be taken in attempting to predict or extrapolate effects in man from effects found in animals. Physical differences (size, shape, fur-bearing, etc.) result in marked differences in the internal field distribution (Kaune & Phillips, 1980), and in different behavioural and homeostatic responses.

With such limited data available on biological effects and interaction mechanisms, the only practical approach left for making a health risk evaluation is to evaluate the available data on exposure levels and effects to determine if thresholds for effects occur (Repacholi, 1984a). In undertaking such an evaluation, it is necessary to be selective as far as the data are concerned. Only reports that provide adequate information on experimental technique and dosimetry should form part of the evaluation. Ideally, from a regulatory viewpoint, only data that have been established and have a direct bearing on health risk should be considered. Publication in a peer reviewed journal helps, but in the final analysis, unless the data have been confidently reproduced, the results should be considered tentative pending confirmation.

It would be ideal to make health risk evaluations on the basis of well-conceived, well-conducted, and well-analysed epidemiological studies. Unfortunately, all such studies on human beings exposed to ELF fields have suffered from one or more deficiencies, as indicated in section 6.

With such a limited scientific data base, the determination of the existence of a true threshold exposure level below which no adverse health effect occurs, cannot be made with confidence. Thus, any health risk analysis for the development of standards must inevitably adopt a phenomenological approach (Kossel, 1982; Repacholi, 1983). In this case, a review of the literature is made to determine the lowest exposure levels at which adverse biological effects have been established. A biological effect that occurs in living organisms or animals may be detected as some general or specific alteration. If the change appears irreversible or pathological, it might be presumed that it could be hazardous to man under comparable exposure conditions. This assumption is made only because insufficient information is available on the effect or the underlying interaction mechanism to make an extrapolation to exposure conditions producing similar effects in human beings and to make a well-substantiated health risk evaluation.

The epidemiological studies (Wertheimer & Leeper, 1979, 1982; Tomenius et al., 1982) suggesting a relationship between childhood or adult cancer and residence in houses at various distances from high current flow due to external electrical wiring configurations, can only be considered as preliminary because of the many criticisms that have been levelled at the studies (section 6).

The studies (Milham, 1982; Wright et al., 1982; Coleman et al., 1983; McDowell, 1983; Vagero & Olin, 1983) suggesting an association between electrical occupations (exposure to electric and magnetic fields) and cancer were analyses of occupational mortality data and subject to many sources of errors (section 6).

Thus, although these reports suggest potential adverse health effects, they cannot be evaluated in terms of health risk until the potentially confounding factors and sources of errors are eliminated. It is of concern, however, that no studies have yet been published following up these reports.

Laboratory studies on human volunteers exposed for short periods to electric fields (up to 20 kV/m) have, in general, shown no effects (Hauf & Wiesinger, 1973; Johansson et al., 1973; Hauf, 1974; Rupilius, 1976; Sander et al., 1982). The results of these studies suggest that no apparent acute effects are likely from exposure to strong electric fields. However, they cannot be used as indicators that no health effects will occur from long-term exposure (months or years).

Studies on the health status of linemen and switch-yard workers have not revealed any differences between exposed and control groups (Knave et al., 1979; Stopps & Janischensky, 1979). As indicated in section 6, these epidemiological studies, although among the more complete, have still suffered from a lack of numbers of persons exposed to high electric field strengths for extended periods. However, these workers are exposed to potentially the highest electric field strengths albeit for short periods of time (section 6, Table 7). These studies do not provide a good data base on which to evaluate the possible health effects from long-term exposure of the general public to electric fields near transmission lines. More definitive information is needed, which in general, can only be provided through both large-scale epidemiological studies and developments in dosimetry that will make it possible to extrapolate the experimental animal results to human beings.

While attempting to arrive at general conclusions concerning the health hazards of ELF electric fields for protection purposes, the fundamental question that requires an answer is whether or not exposure to these electric fields induces any physiological or pathological effects in man.

From a careful review of laboratory studies in vivo and in vitro, and from human studies, the following conclusions can be drawn:

(a) Adverse human health effects from exposure to ELF electric field levels normally encountered in the environment or the workplace have not be established.

(b) Some human beings feel spark discharges in electric fields of about 3 kV/m and perceive the fields between 2 - 10 kV/m. At present, there are no scientific data that suggest that perceiving a field produces an adverse pathological effect.

(c) Exposure to ELF electric fields can alter cellular, physiological, and behavioural events. Although it is not possible to extrapolate these findings to human beings, at present, these studies serve as a warning that unnecessary exposure to electric fields should be avoided.

(d) The preliminary nature of the epidemiological findings on the increased incidence of cancer among children and adults exposed to ELF fields from electric wiring and the relatively small increment in reported incidence, suggest that, although the epidemiological data cannot be dismissed, there must be considerable study before they can serve as useful imputs for risk assessment.

8. STANDARDS AND THEIR RATIONALES

A standard is a general term incorporating both regulations and guidelines and can be defined as a set of specifications or rules to promote the safety of an individual or group of people. A regulation is promulgated under a legal statute and is referred to as a mandatory standard. A guideline generally has no legal force and is issued for guidance only - a voluntary standard. Standards can specify exposure limits and other safety rules for personal exposure, or provide details on the performance, construction, design, or functioning of a device.

To protect the general population and persons occupationally exposed to ELF fields, exposure standards are promulgated. These are basic standards of personnel protection that do not apply to particular devices or equipment, but generally refer to maximum levels to which whole or partial body exposure is permitted from any number of radiation emitting devices. This type of standard normally incorporates safety factors and provides the basic guide for limiting personnel exposure.

To date, few regulatory exposure standards have been promulgated limiting human exposure to ELF fields. Guidelines have been developed in a number of countries, mostly as an interim measure until sufficient information on adverse biological effects becomes available to make some reasonable assessment of health risks, and the exposure levels at which hazards occur.

This section includes a review of all known ELF electric field standards known to the Task Group at the time of publication.

Standards

From a recent review of ELF standards, Repacholi (1984a) found that the greatest interest in regulations or guidelines was in ELF electric fields at power frequencies. With the growth in number and length of high voltage transmission lines, increasing concern has occurred among the public, regulatory agencies, and scientists about possible human health effects from exposure to the electric fields associated with these lines. While there is no definitive evidence of such effects, mounting public fear and activism over hypothesized health risks has caused delays in the licensing and construction of major power transmission facilities, and encouraged the formation of regulatory policy in some countries.

The primary basis for public concern was a series of studies conducted in the USSR in the 1960s (Asanova & Rakov, 1966; Knickerbocker, 1975). These studies resulted in the occupational safety standard in the USSR (1975), which is summerized in Table 11. In addition, a guideline on the design of HV transmission lines near residential areas recommends a limit of 1 kV/m (Lyskov et al., 1975). However, this guideline may be under question (Bourgsdorf, 1980).

Table 11. Electric field exposure limits for workers in installations of 400 kV and higher in the USSR (1975)

Electric-field strength (kV/m)	Permitted exposure duration per day (min)
5	Unrestricted
10	180
15	90
20	10
25	5

Note: 1. If workers are exposed to electric fields of 10kV/m or more for the full time permitted by the standard, they must remain in fields of 5 kV/m or less for the rest of the day.
2. Workers exposed to 10 kV/m or above can remain for the permitted time, provided they are not subject to spark discharges.

The Soviet standard applies to workers in substations or on transmission lines operating at 400 kV and above. The duration of the standard was from 1 January 1977 to 1 January 1982, after which it was to be reviewed and either changed or reaffirmed. At the time of publication of this document, a new standard for electric 50 Hz power frequencies is being discussed by the Council of Mutual Economic Assistance (incorporating Bulgaria, Cuba, Czechoslovakia, the German Democratic Republic, Poland, Romania, and the USSR).

The basis for the Soviet standard is that studies conducted since 1962 on the effects on workers on high-voltage power systems revealed electric field influences on human beings. It is believed that the reaction of the human body to the direct influence of an electrical field is non-specific; it can develop after a comparatively long time (2 - 5 months); it has a long-term consequence, pronounced cumulative effects, and strong dependency on individual physiological peculiarities of the body (Lyskov et al., 1975).

In a design criteria for 1100 kV lines in the USSR, Lyskov et al. (1975) and Bourgsdorf et al. (1976) reported that clearances to ground were determined in order to limit the electric field to 10 - 12 kV/m, at points where the HV transmission lines cross roads, and to 15 - 20 kV/m elsewhere along unpopulated sections of the line routes; a limit of up to 20 kV/m was determined for difficult terrain and hardly accessible areas. These field strengths must not be exceeded at the centre of the span at a height of 1.8 m above the ground and at the lowest sag (at the maximum 15-year temperature).

In the United Kingdom, the National Radiological Protection Board (NRPB, 1982) has issued a proposal for ELF fields. In this consultative document it states: "The Board accepts that exposures to power frequency fields of less than 10 kV/m are safe, although the field may be perceptible at lower values, and that exposures to fields up to 30 kV/m are unlikely to be harmful". The NRPB admits that there is very little information that can be used as a rational basis for limiting exposure and that at 50 Hz, perceptible but harmless effects depend to a large extent on environmental factors and individual sensitivities. However, steps should be taken to prevent such effects from occurring with any degree of regularity. This will generally be achieved if the root mean square field strengths are kept below 10 kV/m. Prolonged exposure to fields greater than 20 kV/m, which induce currents in excess of 0.5 mA in the body, is also undesirable, according to the NRPB.

In Japan, all electric power equipment is subject to the regulation "Technical Practices of Electrical Equipment", an ordinance of the Ministry of International Trade and Industry. The ordinance (Repacholi, 1984a) includes such technical specifications as:

(a) minimum height of electrical conductors;

(b) necessary clearance between a transmission line and building; and

(c) the electrical field strength on the ground surface under the line.

In summary, the ordinance states that the unperturbed electrical field strength 1 m above the ground surface must not exceed 3 kV/m rms. In addition, the line must be built so that it does not pose any risk for human beings. However, in lightly-populated areas such as rice fields, farms, and forests, this limitation is not applied when the line is constructed so that there are no risks for anyone.

A description of the technical basis for this 3 kV/m standard is provided by the Japan IERE Council (1976). The standard is based on the electrostatic induction sensed by a person who has his cheek or finger in contact with the metallic part of the grip of an umbrella.

In Poland (1980), the electromagnetic radiation standard for frequencies from 0.1 - 300 000 MHz, includes a limit on electric field strength at the single frequency of 50 Hz. The standard, effective from 31 January 1980, establishes two "safety" zones. For exposure to 50-Hz electric fields, the zones are:

1st zone (electric fields above 10 kV/m) - prohibited to everyone except workers in electrical substations and personnel working on power lines;

2nd zone (above 1 kV/m to 10 kV/m) - agriculture and recreational activities are allowed, but not the construction of housing, hospitals, schools or kindergartens, except where buildings and farms existed before the regulations were established.

The standard provides details of administrative controls, approval procedures and electromagnetic field measuring authorities. However, no rationale for the values in the standard appear to have been published.

In the USA, there are a number of different standards with regard to the control of electric fields at the edge of RoW (see Glossary for definition) for high-voltage transmission lines. General population and media pressure have prompted public hearings and extensive debate over health effects from these lines. The US Department of Energy, Bonneville Power Administration (BPA) has a criterion on electric field exposure levels that results in a low probability of human perception or annoyance from field effects (Lee et al., 1982). BPA allows a maximum of 9 kV/m on the RoW, when measured 1 m above the ground (Lee et al., 1982). It would seem that the rationale for setting the 9-kV/m level is so that induced body currents in human beings under the lines will not exceed the current permitted by the National Electric Safety Code (5 mA rms).

All 50 states in the USA have some legislation for regulating the safety of the general population in the proximity of transmission lines. Of these, 25 states have enacted legislation requiring the preparation of environmental impact statements for proposed overhead transmission lines with respect to electrical effects. A comprehensive study was completed by the state of New York (1979), in which testimony indicated potential impacts from audible noise and from electrostatic shocks that people can receive when they touch a large vehicle parked under the lines. The testimony failed to demonstrate biological hazards from the field, though further research is necessary to understand better the effects of the fields on biological systems.

Many of the state regulatory agencies have carried out similar studies (Shah, 1979; Montana, 1983) reaching the same basic conclusions as New York (1979). Guidelines from each state on the maximum electric field permitted at the edge of the RoW differ, but are within the range of 1 - 3 kV/m (Table 12). Guidelines for maximum field strength within the RoW varied from 7 to 11 kV/m. Most states comply with the National Electric Safety Code (NESC), which restricts currents in the human body to no more than 5 mA (rms).

Table 12. Recommended electric field levels for high-voltage transmission lines in the USA[a]

State	Max E field (kV/m)		Comments	Reference
	In RoW	Edge RoW		
Minnesota	8	-	Resolution	Shah (1979)
Montana	-	1	Resolution	Montana (1983)
New Jersey	-	3	Resolution	New Jersey (1981)
New York	-	1[b]	Temporar resolution - new EHV lines	New York (1978)
	7	-	Public roads	Shah (1979)
	11	-	Private roads	Shah (1979)
North Dakota	9	-	Resolution	Shah (1979)
Oregon	9	-	State law	Shah (1979)

[a] From: Repacholi (1984a).
[b] 1 kV/m for flat terrain - use 1.6 kV/m as criterion (Sheppard (1983), personal communication).

Note: Most states have adopted NESC (5mA rms).

Only two states in Australia, Victoria and New South Wales, have guidelines for the construction of 500 kV HV transmission lines (Table 13).

In Victoria, the State Electricity Commission designs the 500 kV lines so that the electric field does not exceed 10 kV/m in the RoW or 2 kV/m at the edge of the RoW, when measured 1 m above the ground. Workers in switch-yards are normally restricted to exposures below 10 kV/m, where

Table 13. Guidelines for constructing 500 kV high voltage transmission lines in Australia[a]

State	Max. E field (kV/m)	
	In RoW	Edge RoW
New South Wales[b]	-	2
Victoria	10	2

[a] From: Repacholi (1984a).
[b] Personal communication, Sydney, Australia, Electricity Commission of New South Wales.

practical. The rationale for their guideline, contained in Johnson et al. (1976), was also based on the fact that these values were generally acceptable in many other standards, including the Soviet standard (USSR, 1975).

The Electricity Commission of New South Wales has an internal design standard for 500-kV HVAC lines that states that the electric field strength at the edge of the RoW should not exceed 2 kV/m. However, in practice, the RoW is made sufficiently wide that values of 0.5 kV/m are not exceeded at its edge.

9. PROTECTIVE MEASURES

9.1 Goals

This criteria document does not recommend specific values for electric-field standards, but where a health agency finds that standards are necessary, it provides guidance on the development of standards.

It is understood that standards may be required when it is necessary to ensure that physical agents are not introduced into the environment at levels that may reduce the quality of life. The overall assessment of the impact of electric power on the quality of life involves the balance of positive and negative factors implicit in a cost-benefit analysis. At this time, a cost-benefit analysis cannot be conducted with quantitative precision.

9.2 Groups to be Protected

Protective measures may be considered for electrical utility workers exposed near substations, transformers, capacitors, and circuit breakers or workers exposed near live power transmission or distribution conductors. Depending on the equipment, individual policies and worker/job classifications, the extent of exposures may vary widely, requiring careful review by each affected organization. Workers primarily involved with communications facilities may also be affected. In cases where joint facilities are used (e.g., high-voltage lines near or having common RoWs with low-voltage communications lines), the communications workers may be considered together with electric power utility workers. Workers in industry may also be affected, principally through magnetic field exposures from low-frequency induction heaters and furnaces, large motors, transformers, and similar devices to which personnel are exposed, often at close proximity.

Exposure of the general population occurs during occasional visits to electrical utility facilities, often for recreation in RoWs or, in the case of farmers, for work. Exposures also result from living in the vicinity of a high-voltage transmission line, in the course of using electrical appliances, and generally as an essential aspect of the widespread use of electric power for illumination and power. It should be noted that high-voltage direct current transmission also involves alternating currents as a result of the AC/DC conversion process. These currents occur at several harmonic frequencies in the range below 1 kHz at amplitudes that are much below the level of direct currents. The specific conversion technology and its operational mode must also be considered.

At present, protective measures for the general population are at issue with respect to dwellings located near power-transmission-line corridors. Exposures that originate in the home or home environment are generally weak and exposures to appliance-generated fields are very intermittent. Although they are not thought to be of concern, they have not been closely studied.

9.3 Protection Rationale

Occupational exposures among utility workers have been characterized in data reviewed by Knave et al. (1979) and Male et al. (1982). Relatively few hours are spent in fields at levels above 5 kV/m, in any job. In fields above 10 kV/m, workers are subject to recognised influences of perceptible shock discharges, that reduce worker comfort and increase the possibility of accidents with tools or accidents arising from faulty judgement.

The following protective measures can be taken with regard to workers in fields of about 10 kV/m or more:

(a) the designing of equipment to reduce the likelihood of large potential differences or large current flow between a person and conducting objects;

(b) reduction of daily duration of exposure in proportion to the degree of discomfort experienced; since job assignments, weather, and clothing appear to be major factors, rules can be developed on the basis of practical experience;

(c) use of devices or clothing that reduce the strength of electric fields acting on the body; particular attention should be paid to the protection of linemen working on HV lines with the bare-hand method, when the total residual body current should not exceed values that arise from exposure to external field strengths of less than 10 kV/m.

Electric field exposure up to 20 kV/m, apart from effects due to shocks, is not believed to be an occupational hazard on the basis of information now available. For this reason, protective measures, apart from an altered work schedule, are not suggested in fields below 20 kV/m. Although an occupational hazard is not established in fields above 20 kV/m, as a prudent measure it is suggested that attempts should be made to reduce exposures to levels where no unacceptable discomfort occurs.

In view of the fact that there is no health effect that could be attributed specifically to ELF exposure, it is not practicable to recommend any specific medical examinations, apart from those that may be appropriate for electrical fitters and linemen in general.

GLOSSARY OF TERMS USED IN THE DOCUMENT

ALTERNATING CURRENT: an electric current varying sinusoidally in time.

ALTERNATING ELECTRIC FIELD: the electric field produced by a sinusoidally-oscillating electric charge.

ALTERNATING VOLTAGE: a voltage varying sinusoidally in time.

BIOPHYSICAL: relating to the physical properties of biological systems, e.g., the conductivity of tissue or its permittivity are biophysical quantities.

CIRCADIAN RHYTHM: daily cycle of certain physiological processes such as activity, temperature, and as indicated by the levels of electrolytes, hormones, etc., in body fluids or tissues. More generally, the term refers to a periodic physiological or biochemical change.

CONTROLS: animals, tissues, etc., not subjected to the field or other experimental treatment (see also SHAM-EXPOSED).

CURRENT DENSITY: the flow of electric current across a unit area, a measure of the distribution of current within the object or body tissues measured in amperes per square metre (A/m^2), or microamperes per square centimetre ($\mu A/cm^2$).

EARTH: electrical ground.

EFFECTIVE FIELD: the time-averaged electric field to which a biological system is exposed; this field is less than the unperturbed field because of mutual shielding, e.g., by animals housed as a group.

ELECTRIC FIELD: concept used to represent the force exerted on the unit charge due to the location of electric charges at various sites in a region; the high-voltage-transmission lines electric field is an alternating (50- or 60-Hz) field due to the sinusoidally-oscillating charges located on the conducting wires of the transmission line. Electric fields are capable of performing work on other electric charges moving between points at different potential.

ELECTRIC-FIELD STRENGTH: magnitude of the electric field, measured in volts per metre; (see VOLT PER METRE). The electric-field strength beneath a HV transmission line is generally measured at a fixed height above ground (usually 1 m).

ELF: abbreviation for extremely low frequency.

EXTREMELY LOW FREQUENCY: a frequency between 3 and 300 Hz; but defined in this document as any frequency below 300 Hz.

FARADAY SCREEN: see FARADAY SHIELD CAGE.

FARADAY SHIELD CAGE: grounded cage made of conducting material used to enclose an object subjected to an electric field; the shield, usually composed of metal (eg., copper wire); reduces the electric field strength inside the cage to nearly zero.

FIELD: a region of space in which certain phenomena occur, described by a scalar or vector quantity, the knowledge of which allows the effects of the field to be evaluated.

FREE SPACE: an ideal, perfectly homogeneous medium that possesses relative dielectric and magnetic constants of unity, and in which there is nothing to reflect, refract, or absorb energy. A perfect vacuum possesses these qualities.

GROUND: zero potential, electric earth.

HERTZ (Hz): the unit of frequency for a periodic oscillation corresponding to a complete oscillation per second (ops) or cycle per second (cps).

HIGH TENSION LINE: a high-voltage transmission line.

HORIZONTAL ELECTRIC FIELD: an electric field directed parallel to the Earth's surface; in the laboratory, such fields are created by vertical plates.

HVTL: high-voltage transmission line; typically one operating at or above 345 kV.

IMPEDANCE: the physical property of a material that determines the relation between current flow and potential difference in the material; for direct currents, impedance is identical to resistance; for alternating currents impedance includes the properties of resistance, capacitance, and inductance.

IMPEDANCE TO GROUND: an impedance measured between an object and earth (ground); in caged laboratory animals, this property depends on the caging materials, construction, and electrical design, and the biophysical properties of the animal's footpad; for human beings, skin, clothing, or shoe properties are significant.

INTERNAL ELECTRIC FIELD: electric-field strength measured or calculated for points within the body of an animal or human being exposed to an external electric field.

MAGNETIC FIELD: a concept to describe the force exerted on a unit current produced by moving electrical charges, such as those in an electrical current; the transmission line magnetic field is due to the flow of current in the wires. A magnetic field exerts a force on moving electric charges, such as those in another wire-carrying current or in a moving wire (dynamo principle) always perpendicular to the direction of motion.

MICRO: prefix for 10^{-6}; e.g., microvolt, microampere, micrometre; symbol - μ (Greek letter mu).

MILLI: prefix for 10^{-3}; e.g., millivolt, milliampere; symbol - m.

NANO: prefix for 10^{-9}; symbol - n.

NEUROPHYSIOLOGICAL: relating to the function of the nervous system, e.g., peripheral nerves, the brain, spinal cord, the sub-divisions of those organs and their cellular components, including the nerve fibres.

PHASOR (vector): a phasor is a complex number. It is used in connection with quantities related to the steady alternating state in a linear network or system.

PICO: prefix for 10^{-12}; symbol - p.

PULSE POWER: the power averaged over the duration of a single pulse.

PULSE REPETITION RATE: the rate, usually given in cycles (or pulses) per second, at which pulses are emitted by a pulse system.

PULSE WIDTH: the duration of a pulse in the time interval between the points on the leading and trailing edges.

RIGHT-OF-WAY (RoW): the provision of access to power lines for inspection and maintenance purposes; the concept varies from one country to another. It may take the form of the ownership of land over which the power line passes, or the statutory control of access to this land, or the negotiation of agreements with the landowners. In some countries, the right-of-way applies to a corridor (strip of land), of a certain width, along the transmission line, in which the public access or property rights may be restricted.

rms: root mean square, the square root of the temporal average over a period of the square of the field strength magnitude.

SCALAR: a quantity that is completely specified by a single number.

SCALING: relating an exposure of one animal species to another so that the effect of the electric field can be interpreted on an equal basis; because of shape- and orientation-dependence for both internal and external fields, human beings and animals exposed to the same unperturbed field have very different surface and internal fields.

SHAM-EXPOSED: a control experimental condition in which the animals, tissues, etc., are treated identically to the exposed objects, except that the field or other treatment is not present; distinguished from "controls" by the use of apparatus that is in all ways identical to the exposure apparatus which is not operating.

SPECTRAL CHARACTERISTICS: the frequencies and amplitudes inherent in a particular electric or magnetic field as revealed by a mathematical or experimental technique that "decomposes" the signal into its component frequencies and field strengths (Fourier analysis).

SURFACE ELECTRIC FIELD: the electric field at the outer margin of the object or body; this field is influenced by the shape and configuration of a conducting body and, depending on the degree of curvature, is locally greater than the unperturbed electric field.

TERATOLOGICAL: relating to abnormal anatomy, resulting in deformities, fetal death, still birth, etc., especially in a developing or newborn organism.

UNPERTURBED ELECTRIC FIELD: the field that would exist at the body's location if there were no body located in the electric field. In the case of a uniform field, the field that exists far from the location of a conducting object (such as the human or animal body).

VECTOR: a mathematical-physical quantity that represents a vector quantity - it has magnitude and direction.

VECTOR QUANTITY: any physical quantity in which specifications involve both magnitude and direction and which obeys the parallelogram law of addition.

VERTICAL ELECTRIC FIELD: an electric field directed perpendicular to the Earth's surface; in the laboratory, such fields are created by horizontal electrodes.

VOLT PER METRE: unit of electric field strength; a field of one volt per metre is created in the centre of the midplane of two parallel plates separated by 1 metre and having a potential difference of 1 volt.

REFERENCES

ADEY, W.R. (1975) Evidence for cooperative mechanisms in the susceptibility of cerebral tissue to environmental and intrinsic electric fields. In: Schmitt, F.O., Schneider, D.M., & Crothers, D.M., ed. Functional linkage in biomolecular systems, New York, Raven Press, pp. 325-342.

ADEY, W.R. (1977) Models of membranes of cerebral cells as substrates for information storage. Biosystems, 8: 163-178.

ADEY, W.R. (1980) Frequency and power windowing in tissue interactions with weak electromagnetic fields. Proc. IEEE, 68: 119-125.

ADEY, W.R. (1981) Tissue interactions with non-ionizing electromagnetic fields. Physiol. Rev., 61: 435-514.

ADEY, W.R., BAWIN, S.M., LAWRENCE, A.F., LIN-LIU, S., LUBEN, A.R., LUNDAK, R.L., SAGAN, P.M., & SHEPPARD, A.R. (1981) Tissue interactions with non-ionizing electromagnetic fields, Springfield, Virginia, US Department of Energy (NTIS report DOE/ET/29078-T1).

ALEKSANDROV, M.S., BAKLENEVA, A.M., GLADSTEIN, N.D., OZEROV, V.P., POTAPOV, A.V., & REMIZOV, L.T. (1972) [Fluctuations of the earth's electromagnetic field,] Moscow, Nauka, pp. 195 (in Russian).

ANDERSON, L.E. & PHILLIPS, R.D. (1984) Biological effects of electric fields: an overview. In: Grandolfo, M., Michaelson, S., & Rindi, A., ed. Biological effects and dosimetry of static and ELF electromagnetic fields, New York, Plenum Press.

ANDERSON, L.E., HILTON, D.I., CHESS, E.K., & WILSON, B.W. (1982) Pineal gland response in animals exposed to 60-Hz electric fields. In: Abstracts, Fourth Annual Meeting of the Bioelectromagnetics Society, Los Angeles, California, June-July 1982, p. 15.

ASANOVA, T.P. & RAKOV, A.I. (1966) [The state of health of persons working in electric fields of outdoor 400 and 500 kV switch-yards.] Gig. Tr. Prof. Zabol., 10: 50-52 (in Russian) (translated for IEEE Power Engineering Society, Piscataway, New Jersey, in Special Publication No. 10).

BANKOSKE, J.W., MCKEE, G.W., & GRAVES, H.B. (1976) Ecological influence of electric fields, Palo Alto,

California, Electric Power Research Institute (EPRI Report EA-178, Interim report No. 2).

BARNES, H.C., MCELROY, A.J., & CHRAKOW, J.H. (1967) Rational analysis of electric fields in live-line working. IEEE Trans. Power Appl. Syst., PAS-86: 10-19.

BARONCELLI, P., BATTISTI, S., CHECCUCCI, A., GRANDOLFO, M., SERIO, A., & VECCHIA, P. (1984) [An epidemiological study on the workers of electrical plants: project and research protocol.] In: Proceedings of the XXII National Conference of the Italian Radioprotection Association, pp. 17-20 (in Italian).

BASSETT, A. (1981) Biomedical implications of pulsing electromagnetic fields. In: The Third EBI in vitro Conference, Hasbrouck, New Jersey, June 4-5.

BASSETT, C.A.L. & PAWLUK, R.J. (1974) Acceleration of fracture repair by electromagnetic fields: a surgically non-invasive method. Ann. New York Acad. Sci., 238: 242-262.

BAUCHINGER, M., HAUF, R., SCHMID, E., & DRESP, J. (1981) Analysis of structural chromosome changes and SCE after occupational long-term exposure to electric and magnetic fields from 380 kV-systems. Radiat. environ. Biophys., 19: 235-238.

BAWIN, S.M., KACZMAREK, L.K., & ADEY, W.R. (1975) Effects of modulated VHF fields on the central nervous system. Ann. New York Acad. Sci., 247: 74-80.

BAWIN, S.M., SHEPPARD, A.R., & ADEY, W.R. (1978) Possible mechanisms of weak electromagnetic field coupling in brain tissue. Bioelectrochem. Bioenerg., 5: 67-76.

BAWIN, S.M., SHEPPARD, A.R., MAHONEY, M.D., & ADEY, W.R. (in press) Influence of sinusoidal electric fields on excitability in the rat hippocampal slice. Brain Res.

BENDER, H.A. (1976) A study of the effect of ELF electromagnetic fields upon Drosophila melanogaster, Indiana, University of Notre Dame (Final report, NTIS Document ADA 035956).

BENKOVA, N.P. (1975) The magnetic field of the earth and its variation. In: Physical, mathematical, and biological problems of effects of electromagnetic fields and ionization of air, Moscow, Nauka, pp. 13-24.

BERESNEV, V.K., GUSEV, V.P., ROGATCHEVSKU, B.M., SOLSVEN, I.S., & TOKAREVA, B.G. (1976) [Measurements of fluctuations of the natural electrical field of the earth in the range 1 - 30 m Hz-M: ELF radionoise and its nature,] Rjazan, Medical Institute (in Russian).

BLACKMAN, C.F., ELDER, J.A., WEIL, C.M., BENANE, S.G., EICHINGER, D.C., & HOUSE, D.E. (1979) Induction of calcium-ion efflux from brain tissue by radio-frequency radiation: effects of modulation frequency and field strength. Radio Sci., 14: 93-98.

BLACKMAN, C.F., BENANE, S.G., JOINES, W.T., HOLLIS, M.A., & HOUSE, D.E. (1980) Calcium ion efflux from brain tissue: power density versus internal field-intensity dependencies at tp MHZ RF radiation. Bioelectromagnetics, 1: 277.

BLACKMAN, C.F., BENANE, S.G., KINNEY, L.S., JOINES, W.T., & HOUSE, D.E. (1982) Effects of ELF fields on calcium ion efflux from brain tissue in vitro. Radiat. Res., 92: 510-520.

BLAKEMORE, R.P., FRANKEL, R.B., & WOLFE, R.S. (1979) Ferromagnetism in freshwater bacteria. In: Phillips, R.D., Gillis, M.F., Kaune, W.T., & Mahlum, D.D., ed. Biological effects of extremely low frequency electromagnetic fields. Proceedings of the 18th Annual Hanford Life Sciences Symposium, Richland, Washington, October, 1978, Springfield, Virginia, Technical Information Center, US Department of Energy (DOE Symposium Series 50, NTIS CONF-781016).

BLANCHI, C.L., CEDRINI, L., CERIA, F., MEDA, E., & RE, G. (1973) Exposure of mammalians to strong 50-Hz electric fields. 2. Effects on heart and brain electric activity. Arch. Fisiol., 70: 30-34.

BONNEL, J.A., NORRIS, W.T., PICKLES, J.H., MALE, J.C., & CARTWRIGHT, R.A. (1983) Comments on "Environmental power frequency magnetic fields and suicide". Health Phys., 44: 697-698 (letter to the editor).

BOURGSDORF, M.R. (1980) Round table on UHV feasibility: how the advancement of knowledge has modified the technical-economical feasibility forecasts. Electra, 73: 27-42.

BOURGSDORF, V.V., EMELYIANOV, N.P., LYSKOV, J.I., LIASHENKO, V.S., ROKOTIAN, S.S., & SMIRNOV, B.I. (1976) Design of the EHV 1150 kV AC transmission line. In: International Conference on Large High-Voltage Electric Systems. Proceedings CIGRE Meeting, Paris, Aug. 25 - Sept. 3.

BRACKEN, T.D. (1976) Field measurements and calculations of electrostatic effects of overhead transmission lines. IEEE Trans. Power Appl. Syst., PAS-95: 494-504.

BRIDGES, E.J. (1975) Biological effects of high-voltage electric fields, Palo Alto, California, Electric Power Research Institute, p. 206 (Field Report EPRI 381-1).

BRIDGES, J.E. & FRAZIER, M.J. (1979) The effects of 60 Hertz electric and magnetic fields on implanted cardiac pacemakers, Palo Alto, California (EPRI Report EA 1174).

BROADBENT, D.E., BROADBENT, M.H.P., MALE, J.C., & JONES, M.R.L. (in press) Health of workers exposed to electric fields. Br. J. ind. Med.

BULLOCK, T.H. (1973) Seeing the world through a new sense: electroreception in fish. Am. Sci., 61: 316.

BUSBY, K., DRISCOLL, P.E., & WASHBON, W.E. (1974) A field survey of farmer experience with 765 kV transmission lines, Albany, New York, State Campus (Agricultural Resources Commission Report).

BUTROUS, G.S., MALE, J.C., WEBBER, R.S., BARTON, D.G., MELDRUM, S.J., BONNELL, J.A., & CAMM, A.J. (1983) The effect of power frequency high intensity electric fields on implanted cardiac pacemakers. PACE, 6: 1282-1292.

CABANES, J. & GARY, C. (1981) Direct perception of the electric field. In: International Conference on Large High-Voltage Electric Systems, Stockholm, CIGRE.

CAIN, C.A. (1981) Biological effects of oscillating electric fields: role of voltage-sensitive ion channels. J. Biolectromagn., 2: 23-32.

CARTER, J.H. & GRAVES, H.B. (1975) Effects of high-intensity AC electric fields on the electrocephalogram and electrocardiogram of domestic chicks: literature review and experimental results, University Park, Pennsylvania, Pennsylvania State University.

CERRETELLI, P. & MALAGUTI, C. (1976) Research carried out in Italy by ENEL on the effects of high-voltage electric fields. Rev. gén. Electr., Numéro spécial(juillet): 65-74.

CERRETELLI, P., VEICSTEINAS, A., MARGONATO, V., CANTONE, A., VIOLA, D., MALAGUTI, C., & PREVI, A. (1979) 1000 kV project:

Research on the biological effects of 50 Hz electric fields in Italy. In: Phillips, R.D., Gillis, M.F., Kaune, W.T., & Mahlum, D.D., ed. Biological effects of extremely low frequency electromagnetic fields. Proceedings of the 18th Annual Hanford Life Sciences Symposium, Richland, Washington, October, 1978, Springfield, Virginia, Technical Information Center, US Department of Energy, pp. 241-257 (DOE Symposium Series 50, NTIS CONF-781016).

CHALMERS, J.A. (1967) Atmospheric electricity, 2nd ed., Oxford, Pergamon Press.

CHECCUCCI, A. (1984) An epidemiological investigation of HV substation workers: study design and preliminary results. In: Grandolfo, M., Michaelson, S., & Rindi, A., ed. Biological effects and dosimetry of static and ELF electromagnetic fields, New York, Plenum Press.

CIGRE (1980) Electric and magnetic fields produced by transmission systems - description of phenomena, practical guide for calculation. In: International Conference on Large Voltage Electric Systems, Paris, France, pp. 139.

COATE, W.B. & NEGERBON, W.H. (1970) Insect mutagenesis study M: Project sanguine biological effects test program pilot study, Falls Church, Virginia, Hazelton Laboratories (Final report).

COLEMAN, M., BELL, J., & SKEET, R. (1983) Leukaemia incidence in electrical workers. Lancet, i: 982-983.

CONTI, R., PREVI, A., MARGONATO, V., & VEICSTEINAS, A. (1981) Progress on the research carried out in Italy by ENEL on the effects of high intensity 50 Hz electric fields. In: Proceedings of the CIGRE Symposium 22-81, Paris.

CREIM, J.A., LOVELY, R.H., PHILLIPS, R.D., & KAUNE, W.T. (1980) Test for induction of illness/malaise in rats by exposure to a 60 Hz electric field. Bioelectromagnetics, 1: 241.

DALZIEL, C.F. & LEE, W.R. (1968) Reevaluation of lethal electric currents. IEEE Trans lGA, 4(5): 467-476.

DANILIN, V.A., VORONIN, A.K., & MODORSKI, V.A. (1969) The state of health of personnel working in high-voltage electric fields. Gig. Tr. Prof. Zabol., 13(5): 51-52.

DELORGE, J. (1972) Operant behavior of rhesus monkeys in the presence of extremely low frequency, low intensity magnetic and electric fields, Springfield, Virginia, US Naval Medical Research Laboratory, Experiment 1 (Report NAMRL-1155, NTIS AD 754058).

DELORGE, J. (1973) Operant behaviour of rhesus monkeys in the presence of extremely low frequency, low intensity magnetic fields, Springfield, Virginia, US Naval Medical Research Laboratory (NTIS AD 764532, 1973a; NTIS AD 774106, 1973b).

DELORGE, J. & MARR, M.J. (1974) Operant methods of assessing the effects of ELF electromagnetic fields. In: Persinger, M.A., ed. ELF and VLF electromagnetic field effects, New York, Plenum Press, pp. 145-175.

DENO, D.W. (1974) Calculating electrostatic effects of overhead transmission lines. IEEE Trans. Power Appl. Syst., PAS-93: 1458-1471.

DENO, D.W. (1975) Electrostatic induction formulae. IEEE Trans. Power Appl. Syst., PAS-94: 1524-1536.

DENO, D.W. (1976) Transmission line fields. IEEE Trans. Power Appl. Syst., PAS-95: 1600-1611.

DENO, D.W. (1977) Currents induced in the human body by high-voltage transmission line electric field - measurement and calculation of distribution and dose. IEEE Trans. Power Appl. Syst., PAS-96: 1517-1527.

DENO, D.W. (1979) Monitoring of personnel exposed to a 60 Hz electric field. In: Phillips, R.D., Gillis, M.F., Kaune, W.T., & Mahlum, D.D., ed. Biological effects of extremely low frequency electromagnetic fields. Proceedings of the 18th Annual Hanford Life Sciences Symposium, Richland, Washington, October, 1978, Springfield, Virginia, Technical Information Center, US Department of Energy, pp. 93-108 (DOE Symposium Series 50, NTIS CONF-781016).

DENO, D.W. & ZAFFANELLA, L.E. (1975) Electrostatic effects of overhead transmission lines and stations. In: Transmission line reference book 345 kV and above, Palo Alto, California, Electric Power Research Institute, pp. 248-280 (EPRI Report EL-100-1).

DOLEZALEK, H. (1979) Atmospheric electricity. In: Handbook of chemistry and physics, 50th ed., Boca Raton, Florida, CRC Press, p. F-212.

DUMANSKY, Y.D., POPOVICH, V.M., & KOZYARIN, I.P. (1977) Effects of low frequency (50 Hz) electromagnetic field on functional state of the human body. Gig. i Sanit., 12: 32-35.

DURFEE, W.K., CHANG, R.W., POLK, C., SMITH, L.T., YATES, V.J., PLANTE, P.R., MUTHUKRISHNAN, S., CHEN, H.J., MILLER, L.T., & MARTIN, P.J. (1975) Extremely low frequency electric and magnetic fields effects in domestic birds, Kingston, Rhode Island, University of Rhode Island (Technical report).

ECKERT, E.E. (1977) Sudden unexpected death of infants. Med. klin., 71: 937-941.

EHRET, C.F., GROH, K.R., & RUSSELL, J.J. (1980a) Circadian and ultradian functions in rats exposed to high-voltage electric fields. Bioelectromagnetics, 1: 200.

EHRET, C.F., ROSENBERG, R.S., SACHER, G.A., DUFFY, P.H., GROH, K.R., & RUSSELL, J.J. (1980b) Biomedical effects associated with energy transmission systems: Effects of 60-Hz electric fields on circadian and ultradian physiological and behavioral functions in small rodents, Washington DC, US Department of Energy, Division of Electric Energy Systems (Annual Report).

EISEMANN, B. (1975) [Studies on the long-term effects on man of weak 50 Hz AC currents,] University of Freiberg (Dissertation) (in German).

FAM, W.Z. (1980) Long-term biological effects of very intense 60-Hz electric fields on mice. IEEE Trans. Biomed. Eng., BME-27: 376-381.

FELDSTONE, C.S., POLONIS, J.J., GIBSON, E.G., SMITH, H.D., & DEAN, E.E. (1980) A preliminary study of possible effects of high-intensity 60 Hz electric fields on non-human primate behaviour. Bioelectromagnetics, 1: 200.

FOLE, F.F. (1973) [The HVS effect in electric power substations.] Med. Segur. Trab., 21: 15-18 (in Spanish).

FOLE, F.F., MARTINEZ, F.G., & DUTRUS, E. (1974) New contribution to the study of electromagnetic fields generated by high voltages. Paper presented at AISS Symposium, Paris, March 1974, Chicago, Illinois, Research Institute for Electric Power Research (English translation memorandum E8180-1 by IIT).

FRAZIER, M.E., SAMUEL, J.E. & KAUNE, W.T. (1982) Effects of 60-Hz electric fields on CHO-K1 cells, In: Abstracts, Fourth Annual Meeting of the Bioelectromagnetics Society, Los

Angeles, June-July 1982, Gaithersburg, Maryland, Bioelectromagnetic Society.

FREE, M.J., KAUNE, W.T., PHILLIPS, R.D., & CHENG, H.C. (1981) Endocrinological effects of strong 60 Hz electric fields on rats. Bioelectromagnetics, 2: 105-121.

FRYDMAN, M., LEVY, A., & MILLER, S.E. (1972) Oxidant measurements in the vicinity of energized 765 kV lines. In: IEEE Power Engineering Society, Summer Meeting, San Francisco, California, July, 1982.

FULTON, J.P., COBB, S., PREBLE, L., LEONE, L., & FORMAN, E. (1980) Electrical wiring configurations and childhood leukaemia in Rhode Island. Am. J. Epidemiol., 111: 292-296.

GANN, D.J. (1976) Final report. Electric Power Research Institute, Baltimore, Maryland, John Hopkins University (RP 98-02).

GARY, C. (1976) Effets biologiques d'un champ électrique. Que peut dire l'électricien à ce sujet? Rev. gén. Electr., Numéro spécial(juillet): 5-18.

GAVALAS, R.J., WALTER, D.O., HAMNER, J., & ADEY, W.R. (1970) Effect of low-level, low frequency electric fields on EEG and behaviour in Macaca nemestrina. Brain Res., 18: 491-501.

GAVALAS-MEDICI, R.J. & DAY-MAGDALENO, S.R. (1976) Extremely low frequency, weak electric fields affect schedule-controlled behaviour of monkeys. Nature (Lond.), 261: 256-259.

GOODMAN, E.M., GREENEBAUM, B., & MARRON, M.T. (1976) Effects of extremely low frequency electromagnetic fields on Physarum polycephalum. Radiat. Res., 66: 531-540.

GOODMAN, E.M., GREENEBAUM, B., & MARRON, M.T. (1979) Bioeffects of extremely low-frequency electromagnetic fields. Variation with intensity, waveform, and individual or combined electric and magnetic fields. Radiat. Res., 78(3): 485-501.

GOULD, J.L., KIRSCHVINK, J.L., & DEFEYES, K.S. (1978) Bees have magnetic remanence. Science, 201: 1026-1028.

GRAVES, H.B. (1977) Some biological effects of high intensity, low frequency (60-Hz) electric fields on small birds and mammals. In: Second Symposium and Technical Exhibition on Electromagnetic Compatibility, June 28-30, Montreux, Switzerland.

GRAVES, H.B., CARTER, J.H., KELLMEL, D., & COOPER, L. (1978) Perceptibility and electrophysiological reponse of small birds to intense 60 Hz electric fields. IEEE Trans Power Appl. Syst., PAS-97: 1070-1073.

GRAVES, H.B., LONG, P.D., & POZNANIAK, D. (1979) Biological effects of 60 Hz alternating current fields: a Cheshire cat phenomenon? In: Phillips, R.D., Gillis, M.F., Kaune, W.T., & Mahlum, D.D., ed. Biological effects of extremely low frequency electromagnetic fields. Proceedings of the 18th Annual Hanford Life Sciences Symposium, Richland, Washinton, October, 1978, Springfield, Virginia, Technical Information Center, US Department of Energy, pp. 184-197 (DOE Symposium Series 50, NTIS CONF-781016).

GREENEBAUM, G., GOODMAN, E.M., & MARRON, M.T. (1979a) Effects of extremely low frequency fields on slime mold: studies of electric, magnetic, and combined fields, chromosomenumbers, and other tests. In: Phillips, R.D., Gillis, M.F., Kaune, W.T., & Mahlum, D.D., ed. Biological effects of extremely low frequency electromagnetic fields. Proceedings of the 18th Annual Hanford Life Sciences Symposium, Richland, Washington, October, 1978, Springfield, Virginia, Technical Information Center, US Department of Energy, pp. 117-131 (DOE Symposium Series 50, NTIS CONF-781016).

GREENEBAUM, G., GOODMAN, E.M., & MARRON, M.T. (1979b) Extremely low-frequency fields and the slime mold Physarum polycephalum. Evidence of depressed cellular function and of internuclear interaction. Radio Sci., 14: 103-107.

GREENBERG, B. & BINDOKAS, V.P. (1981) The effects of high-voltage transmission lines on honey bees, Palo Alto, California, Electric Power Research Institute (Report EA-1809).

GREENBERG, B., KUNICH, J.C., & BINDOKAS, V.P. (1979) Effects of high-voltage tranmission lines on honey bees. In: Phillips, R.D., Gillis, M.F., Kaune, W.T., & Mahlum, D.D., ed. Biological effects of extremely low frequency electromagnetic fields. Proceedings of the 18th Annual Hanford Life Sciences Symposium, Richland, Washington, October, 1978, Springfield, Virginia, Technical Information Center, US Department of Energy, pp. 74-84 (DOE Symposium Series 50, NTIS CONF-781016).

GRISSETT, J.D. (1980) Biological effects of electric and magnetic fields associated with ELF communications systems. Proc. IEEE, 68(1): 98-104.

GRODSKY, I.T. (1976) Neuronal membrane: a physical synthesis. Math. Biosci., 28: 191-219.

GUY, A.W., DAVIDOV, S., YANG, G.-Y., & CHOU, C.-K. (1982) Determination of electric current distributions in animals and humans exposed to a uniform 60 Hz high-intensity electric field. Bioelectromagnetics, 3: 47-71.

HANSSON, H.A. (1981a) Purkinje nerve cell changes caused by electric fields: ultrastructural studies on long-term effects on rabbits. Med. Biol., 59: 103-110.

HANSSON, H.A. (1981b) Lamellar bodies in Purkinje nerve cells experimentally induced by electric field. Brain Res., 216: 187-191.

HAUF, G. (1974) [Research on the effects of electrical power industry fields on man,] Munich, Germany, Ludwig Maximillian University (Dissertation) (in German).

HAUF, R. (1974) [Effects of 50 Hz alternating fields on man.] Electrotechn. Z., 26: 381 (in German).

HAUF, R. (1976) [Effects of electromagnetic fields on man.] Electrotechn. Z., 6/7: 181 (in German).

HAUF, R. (1982) Electromagnetic ELF fields. In: Suess, M.J., ed. Non-ionizing radiation protection, Copenhagen, World Health Organization Regional Office for Europe (WHO Regional Publications, European Series No. 10).

HAUF, R. & WIESINGER, J. (1973) Biological effects of technical, electric, and electromagnetic VLF fields. Int. J. Biometeorol., 17: 213-215.

HILTON, D.I. & PHILLIPS, R.D. (1980) Cardiovascular response of rats exposed to 60 Hz electric fields. Bioelectromagnetics, 1: 55-64.

HJERESEN, D.L., KAUNE, W.T., DECKER, J.R., & PHILLIPS, R.D. (1980) Effects of 60 Hz electric fields on avoidance behaviour and activity of rats. Bioelectromagnetics, 1: 299-312.

HJERESEN, D.L., MILLER, M.C., KAUNE, W.T., & PHILLIPS, R.D. (1982) A behavioral response of swine to a 60-Hz electric field. Bioelectromagnetics, 3: 443-451.

HYLTEN-CAVALIUS, N. (1975) Report of the Institute, Quebec, Canada, Institut de Recherche de l'Hydro-Quebec (Report No. IREQ-1160).

IEEE (1978) Committee Report - Measurement of electric and magnetic fields from AC power lines, New York, Institute of Electrical and Electronic Engineers (IEEE, PAS-97, Paper F77591-1).

IEEE (1979) Recommended practices for measurement of electric and magnetic fields from AC power lines, New York, Institute of Electrical and Electronic Engineers (IEEE Standard 6444-1979).

ISSEL, I., KEMPE, H., SEEBER, A., & WOLF, I. (1977) [Occupational-medical and psychological examinations on electrical fitters - comment on a new regulation.] Dtsch Gesundheitswes., 32(33): 1526-1531 (in German).

JAFFE, R.A. (1982) Neurophysical effects in mammals of acute and subchronic exposure to 60-Hz electric fields, Denver, Colorado (Presented at Department of Energy Contractors Review, November).

JAFFE, R.A. (in press) Somatosensory receptors in the paw of cats are stimulated by 60 Hz electric fields. Neurosci. Abstr.

JAFFE, R.A., LASZEWSKI, B.L., CARR, D.B., & PHILLIPS, R.D. (1980) Chronic exposure to a 60-Hz electric field: effects on synaptic transmission and peripheral nerve function in the rat. Bioelectromagnetics, 1: 131-147.

JAFFE, R.A., LASZEWSKI, B.L., & CARR, D.B. (1981) Chronic exposure to a 60 Hz electric field: effects on neuromuscular function in the rat. Bioelectromagnetics, 2: 227-239.

JAHN, H., KUPFER, J., & URBAN, M. (1978) [The efficiency of protective clothing used during high tension work in the German Democratic Republic.] Energietechnik, 28(11): 437-441 (in German).

JAPAN IERE COUNCIL (1976) [Electrostatic induction caused by extra-high-voltage overhead transmission lines,] Japan, IERE Council (in Japanese) (English version in Special document for IERE members No. R-7604).

JOHANSSON, R., LUNDQUIST, A.G., LUNDQUIST, S., & SCUKA, V. (1973) Is there a connection between the electricity in the atmosphere and the function of man? Part III. 50 Hz field variations, Stockholm, Foreign Operations Administration (FOA Report C2621-45; C2627-H5, 1971-73, September).

JOHNSON, J., CONNELLY, K., & SMITH, D. (1976) Influence of electric field effects on 500 kV system design, Paris, Conference Internationale des Grands Reseaux Electriques (CIGRE Paper 31.05).

KALMIJN, A.J. (1966) Electroperception in sharks and rays. Nature (Lond.), 212: 1232-1233.

KAUNE, W.T. & GILLIS, M.F. (1981) General properties of the interaction between animals and ELF electric fields. Bioelectromagnetics, 2: 1-11.

KAUNE, W.T. & PHILLIPS, R.D. (1980) Comparison of the coupling of grounded humans, swine, and rats to vertical, 60-Hz electric fields. Bioelectromagnetics, 1: 117-130.

KAUNE, W.T., HJERESEN, D.L., RICHARDSON, R.L., & BEAMER, J.L. (1978) A method for the exposure of miniature swine to vertical 60 Hz electric fields. IEEE Trans. Biomed. Eng., BE-25: 276-283.

KAUNE, W.T., ALLEN, C.H., & BEAMER, J.L. (1980) Biological effects of 60 Hz electric fields on miniature swine. IEEE Trans. Power Appl. Syst., PAS-99: 120.

KLEIMENOVA, N.G. (1963) [Current concepts on the nature of high-frequency variations of the earth's electromagnetic field.] Izv. AV SSSR, 12: 1798-1813 (in Russian).

KNAVE, B. (1984) Epidemiological studies on effects of exposure to ELF electromagnetic fields. In: Grandolfo, M., Michaelson, S., & Rindi, A., ed. Biological effects and dosimetry of static and ELF electromagnetic fields, New York, Plenum Publishing Corporation.

KNAVE, B., GAMBERALE, F., BERGSTROM, S., BIRKE, E., IREGREN, A., KOLMODIN-HEDMAN, B., & WENNBERG, A. (1979) Long-term exposure to electric fields. A cross-sectional epidemiological investigation on occupationally-exposed high-voltage substations. Scand. J. Work Environ. Health, 5: 115-125.

KNICKERBOCKER, G.G. (1975) Study in the USSR of medical effects of electric fields of electric power systems, New York, Institute of Electrical and Electronic Engineers Power Engineering Society (Special Publication No. 10).

KNICKERBOCKER, G.G., KOUWENHOVEN, W.B., & BARNES, H.C. (1967) Exposure of mice to a strong AC electric field: an experimental study. IEEE Trans. Power Appl. Syst., PAS-86(4): 498-505.

KOROBKOVA, V.P., MOROZOV, Y.A., STOLAROV, M.S., & YAKUB, Y.A. (1972) Influence of electric field in 500 and 750 kV switch-yards on maintenance staff and means for its protection. In: International Conference on Large High Tension Electric Systems, Paris, 28 August (CIGRE 23-06).

KOSSEL, F. (1982) Regulations and enforcements procedures. In: Suess, M.J., ed. Non-ionizing radiation protection, Copenhagen, World Health Organization, Regional Office for Europe (WHO Regional Publications, European Series No. 10).

KOTTER, F.R. & MISAKIAN, M. (1977) AC transmission line field measurements, Springfield, Virginia, National Technical Information Service (Prepared for US Department of Energy NBS report No. HCP/T-6010/E1).

KOUWENHOVEN, W.B., LANGWORTHY, O.R., SINGEWALD, M.L., & KNICKERBOCKER, G.G. (1967) Medical evaluation of man working in AC electric fields. IEEE Trans. Power Appl. Syst., PAS-8: 506-511.

KRASNOGORSKAJA, N.V. & REMIZOV, V.P. (1975) [Pulsations of the earth's electric field.] In: Physico-mathematical and biological problems of effects of electromagnetic fields and ionization of air, Moscow, Nauka, pp. 49-56 (in Russian).

KRIVOVA, T.E., LUKOVKIN, V.V., & SAZANOVA, T.E. (1973) Influence of the electric field of industrial frequency and discharges on the human organism. In: Filippov, V. & Morozov, J.A., ed. Protection against the effects of the electro-magnetic fields and electric current in industry, Moscow, The All-Union Research Institute for Labor Protection, pp. 16-22.

KRUEGER, A.P. & REED, E.J. (1975) A study of the biological effects of certain ELF electromagnetic fields. Int. J. Biometeorol., 19: 194-201.

KRUEGER, A.P., CIAROLA, A.J., BRADLEY, J.W., & SHREKERHAMER, A. (1975) Effects of electromagnetic fields on fecundity in chickens. Ann. New York Acad. Sci., 247: 391-400.

KRUMPE, P.E. & TOCKMAN, M.S. (1974) Evaluation of the health of personnel working near Project Sanguine Beta Test Facility from 1971-72. In: Llaurado, J., Sances, A., & Battocletti,

J.H., ed. Biologic and clinical effects of low frequency magnetic and electric fields, Springfield, Illinois, Charles C. Thomas.

KUPFER, J. (1979) [A curve for limiting the occurrence of cardiac fibrillation induced by 50 Hz current.] Elektrie, 33(11): 608-609 (in German).

KUPFER, J. (1982) [Investigation to the heart fibrillation - threshold at 50 Hz alternating current.] Elektro-Prakt., 36(11): 387-390 (in German).

KUPFER, J. & ISSEL, F. (1975) [Protective measures and occupational-medical criteria for work under live-line conditions.] Energietechnik, 25(8): 352-353 (in German).

KUPFER, J., BASTEK, R., & EGGERT, S. (1981) [Critical values in connection with fatal accidents involving electric current.] Z. ges. Hyg., 27(1): 9-12 (in German).

LAMBDIN, J.D. (1978) A comparison of measurement techniques to determine electric fields and magnetic flux under EHV overhead power transmission lines, Las Vegas, Nevada, US Environmental Protection Agency (ORP/EAD 78-1).

LEBARS, H. & ANDRE, G. (1976) Biological effects of an electric field on rats and rabbits. Rev. gén. Electr., Numéro spécial(juillet): 91-97.

LEBARS, H., ANDRE, G., PUPIN, F., & LABIE, CH. (1983) Les effets biologiques des champs électriques - effets sur le rat, le souris, le cobaye. Rec. Méd. vét., 159(10): 823-837.

LEE, J.M., BRACKEN, T.D., & ROGERS, L.E. (1979) Electric and magnetic fields as considerations in environmental studies of transmission lines. In: Phillips, R.D., Gillis, M.F., Kaune, W.T., & Mahlum, D.D., ed. Biological effects of extremely low frequency electromagnetic fields. Proceedings of the 18th Annual Hanford Life Sciences Symposium, Richland, Washington, October, 1978, Springfield, Virginia, Technical Information Center, US Department of Energy, pp. 55-73 (DOE Symposium Series 50, NTIS CONF-781016).

LEE, J.M., BRUNKE, J.H., LEE, G.E., REINER, G.L., & SHON, F.L. (1982) Electrical and biological effects of transmission lines: a review, Portland, Oregon, US Department of Energy, Bonneville Power Administration, p. 93.

LOVELY, R.H. (1982) Neurobehavioural effects in rats of acute and subchronic exposure to 60 Hz electric fields. Presented at Department of Energy Contractor's Review, Denver, Colorado, November.

LOVSTRAND, K.G., LUNDQUIST, S., BERGSTROM, S., & BIRKE, E. (1979) Exposure of personnel to electric fields in Swedish extra-high-voltage substations: field strength and dose measurements. In: Phillips, R.D., Gillis, M.F., Kaune, W.T., & Mahlum, D.D., ed. Biological effects of extremely low frequency electromagnetic fields. Proceedings of the 18th Annual Hanford Life Sciences Symposium, Richland, Washington, October, 1978, Springfield, Virginia, Technical Information Center, US Department of Energy, pp. 85-92 (DOE Symposium Series 50, NTIS CONF-781016).

LUBEN, A.R., CAIN, C.JD., CHI-YUN CHEN, M., ROSEN, D.M., & ADEY, W.R. (1982) Effects of electromagnetic stimuli on bone and bone cells in vitro: inhibition of responses to parathyroid hormone by low-energy, low-frequency fields. Proc. Natl Acad. Sci., 79: 4180-4184.

LYLE, D.B., SCHECTER, P., ADEY, W.R., & LUNDAK, R.L. (1983) Suppression of T-lymphocyte cytotoxicity following exposure to sinusoidally amplitude modulated HF fields. Bioelectromagnetics, 4: 281-292.

LYMANGROVER, J.R., KEKN, E., & SETO, Y.J. (1983) 60-Hz electric field alters the steriodogenic response of rat adrenal tissue, in vitro. Life Sci., 32: 691-696.

LYSKOV, Y.I., EMMA, YU.S., & STOLYAROV, M.D. (1975) The factors of electrical field that have an influence on a human. In: Three russian papers on EHV/UHV transmission line and substation design, Boston, Massachusetts, Charles T. Main, Inc.

MALBOYSSON, E. (1976) Medical control of men working within electrical fields. Rev. gén. Electr., Numéro spécial(juillet): 75-80.

MALE, J.C., MINORS, R.H., & NORRIS, W.T. (1982) Exposure of power transmission and distribution staff to 50 Hz electric fields: a measurement survey. In: 4th Annual Meeting of the Bioelectromagnetics Society, Los Angeles, June-July, 1982 (Abstract A-7).

MANDERS, A.H.E. & VAN NIELEN, N.S. (1981) [The magnetic field surrounding high tension lines in the Netherlands and their influence on humans and animals.] Elektrotechniek, 59: 7 (in Dutch).

MANTELL, B. (1975) [Investigations into the effects on man of an alternating magnetic field at 50 Hz,] University of Freiburg (Dissertation) (in German).

MARINO, A.A. & BECKER, R.O. (1977) Biological effects of extremely low frequency electric and magnetic fields: a review. Physiol. Chem. Phys., 9: 131-147.

MARINO, A.A., BERGER, T.J., MITCHELL, J.T., BAHACEK, B.A., & BECKER, R.O. (1974) Electric field effects in selected biologic systems. Ann. New York Acad. Sci., 238: 436-444.

MARINO, A.A., BERGER, T.J., AUSTIN, B.P., BECKER, R.O., & HART, R.X. (1976) Evaluation of electrochemical information transfer system. I. Effect of electric fields on living organisms. J. Electrochem. Soc., 123: 1199-1200.

MARINO, A.A., CULLEN, J.M., REICHMANIS, M., & BECKER, R.O. (1979) Power frequency electric fields and biological stress: a cause effect relationship. In: Phillips, R.D., Gillis, M.F., Kaune, W.T., & Mahlum, D.D., ed. Biological effects of extremely low frequency electromagnetic fields. Proceedings of the 18th Annual Hanford Life Sciences Symposium, Richland, Washington, October, 1978, Springfield, Virginia, Technical Information Center, US Department of Energy, pp. 258-276 (DOE Symposium Series 50, NTIS CONF-781016).

MARINO, A.A., REICHMANIS, M., BECKER, R.O., ULLRICH, B., & CULLEN, J.M. (1980) Power frequency electric field induces biological changes in successive generations of mice. Experientia (Basel), 36(3): 309-311.

MARRON, M.T., GOODMAN, E.M., & GREENBAUM, B. (1975) Mitotic delay in the slime mould Physarum polycephalum induced by low intensity 60- and 75-Hz electromagnetic fields. Nature (Lond.), 254: 66-67.

MATHEWSON, N.S., OOSTA, G.M., & LEVIN, S.G. (1977) Extremely low frequency (ELF) vertical electric field exposure of rats: search for growth, food consumption, and blood metabolite alterations, Bethesda, Maryland, Armed Forces Radiobiology Research Institute Defense Nuclear Agency (Final Report No. X5B09).

MCCLANAHAN, B.J. & PHILLIPS, R.D. (1983) The influence of electric field exposure on bone growth and fracture repair in rats. Bioelectromagnetics, 4: 11-20.

MCDOWALL, M.E. (1983) Leukaemia mortality in electrical workers in England and Wales. Lancet, 8318: 246.

MILHAM, S. (1982) Mortality from leukaemia in workers exposed to electrical and magnetic fields. New Engl. J. Med., 307: 249.

MILLER, C.J. (1967) The measurements of electric fields in live line working. IEEE Trans. Power Appl. Syst., PAS-85: 493-498.

MILLER, D.A. (1974) Electric and magnetic fields produced by commercial power systems. In: Llaurado, J., Sances, A., & Battocletti, J.H., ed. Biologic and clinical effects of low frequency magnetic and electric fields, Springfield, Illinois, Charles C. Thomas, pp. 62-70.

MILLER, M.W. (1980) Letter to the editor re "Electrical wiring configurations and childhood cancer". Am. J. Epidemiol., 112(1): 165-168.

MILLER, M.W., CARSTENSEN, E.L., KAUFMAN, G.E., & ROBERTSON, D. (1979) 60-Hz electric field parameters associated with the perturbation of a eukaryotic system. In: Phillips, R.D., Gillis, M.F., Kaune, W.T., & Mahlum, D.D., ed. Biological effects of extremely low frequency electromagnetic fields. Proceedings of the 18th Annual Hanford Life Sciences Symposium, Richland, Washington, October, 1978, Springfield, Virginia, National Technical Information Service, US Department of Energy, pp. 109-116 (DOE Symposium Series 50, NTIS CONF-781016).

MITTLER, S. (1972) Low frequency electromagnetic radiation and genetic aberrations. Final Report, Springfield, Virginia, National Technical Information Service, Northern Illinois University (Report No. AD-749959).

MONTANA (1983) Preferred and alternative routes for the Bonneville Power Administrations 500 kV line from Garrison-West, Helena, Montana, Bonneville Power Administrations.

MOOS, W.S. (1964) A preliminary report on the effects of electric fields on mice. Aerosp. Med., 35: 374-377.

MORRIS, J.E. & PHILLIPS, R.D. (1982) Effects of 60 Hz electric fields on specific humoral and cellular components of the immune system. Bioelectromagnetics, 3: 341-312.

MORRIS, J.E. & PHILLIPS, R.D. (1983) Effects of 60-Hz electric fields on specific humoral and cellular components of the immune systems. Bioelectromagnetics, 4: 294.

NEW JERSEY (1981) Minutes of the Commission on Radiation Protection, New Jersey, Department of Environmental Health (February 18).

NEW YORK (1979) Potential environmental effects of 765 kV transmission lines. Views before the New York State Public Service Commission, Cases 26529 and 26559, Washington DC, US Department of Energy, Environmental Control Technology Division.

NORDSTROM, S. & BIRKE, E. (1979) Investigation into genetic risks for employees of Swedish power companies exposed to electric fields from 400 kV, Umea, Sweden, University of Umea, Department of Medical Genetics, pp. 1-30.

NORDSTROM, S., BIRKE, E., GUSTAVSSON, L., & NORDENSON, I. (1981) [Workers in high tension steel works - a study of the outcome of pregnancy and chromosome fracture,] Sweden, University of Umea (in Swedish).

NORDSTROM, S., BIRKE, E., & GUSTAVSSON, L. (1983) Reproductive hazards among workers at high-voltage substations. Bioelectromagnetics, 4: 91-101.

NOVAL, J.J., SOHLER, A., REISBERG, R.B., COYNE, H., STRAUB, K.D., & MCKINNEY, H. (1976) Extremely low frequency electric field induced changes in rate of growth of brain and liver enzymes of rats, Pennsylvania, Temple University School of Medicine (NTIS Document ADA 035959).

NRPB (1982) Health protection of workers and members of the general public against the dangers of extra low frequency, radiofrequency, and microwave radiations: a consultative proposal, Chilton, Didcot, England, National Radiological Protection Board (OX11ORQ).

PEARSONS, K.S., BENNET, R.L., & FIDEL, S.A. (1979) Initial study on the effects of transformer and transmission line noise on people, Vol. 1: annoyance, Vol. 2: sleep interference, Vol. 3: community reaction, Palo Alto, California, Electrical Power Research Institute (EPRI EA 1240).

PERRY, F.S., REICHMANIS, M., MARINO, A.A., & BECKER, R.O. (1981) Environmental power frequency magnetic fields and suicide. Health Phys., 41: 267-277.

PHILLIPS, R.D. (1981) Biological effects of 60 Hz electric fields on small and large animals. In: Biological effects of static and low frequency electromagnetic fields. Symposium of the US/USSR Scientific Exchange Program on Physical Factors, Kiev, USSR, May 4-8, Kiev, USSR, A.N. Muszeer Research Institute of General and Commercial Hygiene (in Russian).

PHILLIPS, R.D. (1983) Biological effects of electric fields on miniature pigs. In: Proceedings of the Fourth Workshop of the US/USSR Scientific Exchange on Physical Factors in the Environment, June 21-24 1983, Research Triangle Park, North Carolina, National Institute of Environmental Health Sciences.

PHILLIPS, R.D., GILLIS, M.F., KAUNE, W.T., & MAHLUM, D.D., ed. (1979) In: Biological effects of extremely low frequency electromagnetic fields. Proceedings of the 18th Annual Hanford Life Sciences Symposium, Richland, Washington, October, 1978, Springfield, Virginia, Technical Information Center, US Department of Energy, pp. 577 (DOE Symposium Series 50, NTIS CONF-781016).

PHILLIPS, R.D., ANDERSON, L.E. & KAUNE, W.T. (1981) Biological effects of high strength electric fields on small laboratory animals, Washington DC, US Department of Energy, Division of Electric Energy Systems (DOE/RL01830/T7).

PILLA, A.A. (1980) Electrochemical information transfer and its possible role in the control of cell function. In: Brighton, C.T., ed. Electric and magnetic control of musculoskeletal growth and repair, New York, Grune and Stratton.

PILLA, A.A. & MARGULES, G.S. (1977) Dynamic interfacial electrochemical phenomena at living cell membranes: application to the toad urinary bladder membrane system. J. Electrochem. Soc., 124(11): 1697-1707.

PILWAT, G., RICHTER, H.P., & ZIMMERMANN, U. (1981) Giant culture cells by electric field-induced fusion. FEBS Lett., 133: 169-174.

POHL, H.A. (1978) Dielectrophosesis: the behaviour of matter in non-uniform electric fields, London, Cambridge University Press.

POLAND (1980) Specific requirements for basic safety to protect against electromagnetic non-ionizing radiation harmful to people and their environment, Warsaw, Polish Peoples Republic, pp. 277-278 (Gazette of Current Legislation No. 25).

POLK, C. (1974) Sources, propagation, amplitude, and temporal variation of extremely low frequency (0 - 100 Hz) electromagnetic fields. In: Llaurado, J.G., Sances, A., & Battocletti, J.H., ed. Biologic and clinical effects of low frequency magnetic and electric fields, Springfield, Illinois, Charles C. Thomas, pp. 21-48.

PORTET, R.T. (1983) Study of the thyroid and surrenal glands into rats chronically exposed to a heavy electrical field. C. R. Séance Soc. Biol. Fil., 117(3): 290.

PORTET, R.T., CABANES, J., PERRE, J., & DELOST, N. (in press) Développement du jeune lapin soumis à un champ électrique intense. C. R. Séance Soc. Biol. Fil.

POZNANIAK, D.T., JOHNSON, J.G., MCKEE, G.W., & GRAVES, H.B. (1979) The design of exposure systems for studying the biological effects of 60 Hz electric fields on small plants and animals. In: Phillips, R.D., Gillis, M.F., Kaune, W.T., & Mahlum, D.D., ed. Biological effects of extremely low frequency electromagnetic fields. Proceedings of the 18th Annual Hanford Life Sciences Symposium, Richland, Washington, October, 1978, Springfield, Virginia, Technical Information Center, US Department of Energy, pp. 159-171 (DOE Symposium Series 50, NTIS CONF-781016).

PRESMAN, A.S. (1971) [Electromagnetic fields in the biosphere,] Moscow, Znane, pp. 64 (in Russian).

RAGAN, H.A., BUSCHBOM, R.L., PIPES, M.J., PHILLIPS, R.D., & KAUNE, W.T. (1983) Hematologic and serum chemistry studies in rats exposed to 60-Hz electric fields. Bioelectromagnetics, 4(1): 79-90.

REICHMANIS, M., PERRY, F.S., MARINO, A.A., & BECKER, R.O. (1979) Relation between suicide and the electromagnetic field of overhead power lines. Physiol. Chem. Phys., 11: 403.

REPACHOLI, M.H. (1983) Differentiation between biological effects and health hazards: scaling from animals. In: Grandolfo, M., Michaelson S., & Rindi, A., ed. Biological effects and dosimetry of non-ionizing radiation, New York, Plenum Press.

REPACHOLI, M.H. (1984a) Health risk assessment of static and ELF electric and magnetic fields. In: Grandolfo, M., Michaelson, S., & Rindi, A., ed. Biological effects and dosimetry of static and ELF electromagnetic fields, New York, Plenum Publishing Corporation (in press).

REPACHOLI, M.H. (1984b) Standards on static and ELF electric and magnetic fields and their scientific basis. In: Grandolfo, M., Michaelson, S., & Rindi, A., ed. Biological effects and dosimetry of static and ELF electromagnetic fields, New York, Plenum Publishing Corporation (in press).

REVNOVA, N.V., AZANOVA, T.P., & SEMENOVSKAYA, N.A. (1968) Effects of the high-intensity electric field of industrial frequency. In: Proceedings of the All-Union Symposium on the Hygiene of Labour and Biological Effects of the Radiofrequency Electromagnetic Waves.

RICHTER, H.P., SCHEURICH, P., & ZIMMERMANN, U. (1981) Electric field-induced fusion of sea urchin eggs. Dev. Growth Differ., 23: 479-486.

ROACH, J.F., CHARTIER, V.L., & DIETRICH, F.M. (1973) Experimental oxidant production rates for EHV transmission lines and theoretical estimates of ozone concentrations near operating lines. In: IEEE Power Engineering Society, Summer Meeting, Vancouver, Canada, July 1973.

ROBERGE, P.F. (1976) Study on the state of health of electrical maintenance workers on Hydro-Quebec 735 kV power transmission system, Montreal, Quebec, Canada, Institut de Recherche de l'Hydro-Quebec (Final report).

ROSENBERG, R.S., DUFFY, P.H., SACHER, G.A., & EHRET, C.F. (1983) Relationship between field strength and arousal response in mice exposed to 60-Hz electric fields. Bioelectromagnetics, 4: 181-191.

RUPILIUS, J.P. (1976) [Investigations on the effects on man of an electrical and magnetic 50-Hz alternating field,] Freiberg, Germany, Albert Ludwig University (Dissertation) (in German).

SAGAN, P.M., STELL, M., & ADEY, W.R. (1981) Absolute threshold sensitivity of rats to 60 Hz electric fields. In: Third Annual Meeting of the Bioelectromagnetics Society, August, Washington DC (Abstract).

SANDER, R., BRINKMANN, J., & KUHNE, B. (1982) Laboratory studies on animals and human beings exposed to 50 Hz electric and magnetic fields. In: International Congress on Large High-Voltage Electric Systems, September 1-9, Paris (Paper 36-01).

SAVIN, B.M., SHANDALA, M.G., NIKONOVA, K.V., & MOROZOV, YU.A. (1978) Methods for studying and criteria for evaluating the biological effects of electric fields of industrial frequency. In: American-Soviet Symposium on Superhigh Supply Lines, May, Tashkent.

SAZONOVA, T.E. (1967) Physiological and hygienic assessment of labour conditions at 400 - 500 kV outdoor switch-yards, Profizdat, Institute of Labour Protection of the All-Union Central of Trade Unions (Scientific Pubs. Issue 46); 1975, Piscataway, New Jersey, IEEE Power Engineering Society (Translation in Special Publication No. 10.).

SCHNEIDER, R.P. & KAUNE, W.T. (1981) The effect of 60 Hz electric fields on virus-induced leukaemia in chickens. In: Biological effects of high-strength electric fields on small laboratory animals, Washington DC, Electric Energy Systems Division, Department of Energy (Interim Report July 1981, DOE/RL/01830-T7).

SCHWAN, H.P. (1977) Electrical membrane potentials, tissue excitation, and various relevant interpretations. In: Biologic effects of electric and magnetic fields associated with proposed project seafarer, Washington DC, National Academy of Sciences.

SCHWAN, H.P. (1982a) Nonthermal cellular effects of electromagnetic fields: AC-field induced ponderomotoric forces. Br. J. Cancer, 45(Suppl. V): 220-224.

SCHWAN, H.P. (1982b) Biophysics of the interaction of electromagnetic energy with cells and membranes. In: Grandolfo, M., Michaelson, S., & Rindi, A., ed. Biological effects and dosimetry of non-ionizing radiation, New York, Plenum Press.

SETO, Y.J., LYMANGROVER, J.R., DUNLAP, W.P., HSIEH, S.T., & MAJEAU-CHARGOIS, D. (1982) Some endocrine effects on rats with chronic exposure to 80 kV/m field for three generations. In: Abstracts, Fourth Annual Meeting of the Bioelectromagnetics Society, Los Angeles, CA, June-July 1982, Gaithersburg, MD, Bioelectromagnetics Society.

SHAH, K.R. (1979) Review of state/federal environmental regulations pertaining to the electrical effects of overhead transmission lines: 1978, Springfield, Virginia, US Department of Energy (Publication HCP/EV-1802).

SHEPPARD, A.R. (1983) Biological effects of high-voltage AC transmission lines, Springfield, Virginia, NTIS (Report to the Montana Department of Natural Resources and Conservation, No. P.B. 83 207241).

SHEPPARD, A.R. & ADEY, W.R. (1979) The role of cell surface polarization in biological effects of extremely low frequency fields. In: Phillips, R.D., Gillis, M.F., Kaune, W.T., & Mahlum, D.D., ed. Biological effects of extremely low frequency electromagnetic fields. Proceedings of the 18th Annual Hanford Life Sciences Symposium, Richland, Washington, October, 1978, Springfield, Virginia, Technical Information Center, US Department of Energy, pp. 147-158 (DOE Symposium Series 50, NTIS CONF-781016).

SHEPPARD, A.R. & EISENBUD, M. (1977) Biologic effects of electric and magnetic fields of extremely low frequency, New York, New York University Press.

SHEPPARD, A.R., FRENCH, E., & ADEY, W.R. (1980) ELF electric fields alter neuronal excitability in Aplysia neurons. Bioelectromagnetics, 1: 227 (Abstract).

SHIH, C.H. & DIPLACIDO, J. (1980) The extent of ELF radiation from high-voltage transmission lines. In: Meeting of the Bioelectromagnetics Society, September, San Antonio, Texas (Abstract 135).

SIKOV, M.R., MONTGOMERY, L.D., & SMITH, L.G. (1979) Developmental toxicology studies with 60 Hz electric fields. In: Phillips, R.D., Gillis, M.F., Kaune, W.T., & Mahlum, D.D., ed. Biological effects of extremely low frequency electromagnetic fields. Proceedings of the 18th Annual Hanford Life Sciences Symposium, Richland, Washington, October, 1978, Springfield, Virginia, Technical Information Center, US Department of Energy, pp. 335-347 (DOE Symposium Series 50, NTIS CONF-781016).

SIKOV, M.R., PHILLIPS, R.D., & BUSCHBOM, R.L. (1982) Effects of exposure to 60-Hz electric fields on the development of Hanford miniature swine. Teratology, 25: 76a.

SILNEY, J. (1979) [Effects of electric fields on the human organism,] Cologne, Institut zur Erforschung elektrischer Unfälle, pp. 39 (Medizinisch-Technischer Bericht) (in German).

SINGEWALD, M.L., LANGWORTHY, O.R., & KOUWENHOVEN, W.B. (1973) Medical follow-up study of high-voltage linemen working in AC electric fields. IEEE Trans. Power Appl. Syst., PAS-92: 1307-1309.

SPIEGEL, R.J. (1977) Magnetic coupling to a prolate spheroid model of man. IEEE Trans. Power Appl. Syst., PAS-96(1): 208-212.

SPIEGEL, R.J. (1981) Numerical determination of induced currents in humans and baboons exposed to 60 Hz electric fields. IEEE Trans. EMC, EMC-23: 382-390.

STERN, S., LATIES, V.G., STANCAMPIANO, C., & DELORGE, J.O. (1980) Detection of 60 Hz electric fields by rats: preliminary results. Bioelectromagnetics, 1: 243.

STERN, S., LATIES, V.G., STANCAMPIANO, C., COX, C., & DELORGE, J.O. (1983) Behavioural detection of 60 Hz electric fields by rats. Bioelectromagnetics, 4: 215-247.

STOPPS, G.J. & JANISCHEWSKY, W. (1979) Epidemiological study of workers maintaining HV equipment and transmission lines in Ontario, Vancouver, BC, Canadian Electrical Association.

STRUMZA, M.V. (1970) Influence sur la santé humaine de la proximité des conducteurs de l'électricité à haute tension. Arch. Mal. prof., 31: 269-276.

TAKAGI, T. & MUTO, T. (1971) Influences upon human bodies and animals of electrostatic induction caused by 500 kV transmission lines, Tokyo, Japan, Tokyo Electric Power Company.

TAKASHIMA, S., ONORAL, B., & SCHWAN, H.P. (1979) Effects of modulated RF energy on the EEG of mammalian brains. Radiat. environ. Biophys., 16: 15-27.

TELL, R.A. (1983) Instrumentation for measurement of radiofrequency electromagnetic fields: equipment, calibrations, and selected applications. In: Grandolfo, M., Michaelson, S., & Rindi, A., ed. Biological effects and dosimetry of non-ionizing radiation, radiofrequency and microwave energies, New York, Plenum Press.

TENFORDE, T.S. (1980) Thermal aspects of electromagnetic field interactions with bound calcium ions at the nerve cell surface. J. theor. Biol., 83: 517-521.

TOMENIUS, L., HELLSTROM, L., & ENANDER, B. (1982) Electrical constructions and 50 Hz magnetic field at the dwellings of tumour cases (0 - 18 years of age) in the county of Stockholm. In: Proceedings of the International Symposium on Occupational Health and Safety in Mining and Tunneling, June 21-25, Prague.

TRANSMISSION LINE REFERENCE BOOK (1975) 345 kV and above, Palo Alto, California, Electric Power Research Institute.

USSR (1975) Occupational safety standards system. Electrical fields of current industrial frequency of 400 kV and higher. General safety requirements. GOST Stand. (Moscow), 12(1): 2-75.

UTIDJIAN, H.M.D. (1979) Feasibility of an epidemiological study of workers occupationally-exposed to high-voltage electric fields in the electric power industry, Palo Alto, California, Electric Power Research Institute (Final report EPRI EA-1020).

VAGERO, D. & OLIN, R. (1983) Incidence of cancer in the electronics industry: using the new Swedish Cancer Environment Registry as a screening instrument. Br. J. ind. Med., 40: 188-192.

VANJAN, L.P. (1975) [On the magnetospheric-ionospheric components of atmospheric electric field.] In: Physico-mathematical and biological problems of electromagnetic field effects and air ionization. Proceedings of the All-Soviet Scientific Symposium, November 25-27, Yalta, Moscow, Nauka, Vol. 1, pp. 48-49 (in Russian).

WACHTEL, H. (1979) Firing pattern changes and transmembrane currents produced by extremely low frequency fields in pacemaker neurons. In: Phillips, R.D., Gillis, M.F., Kaune, W.T., & Mahlum, D.D., ed. Biological effects of extremely low frequency electromagnetic fields. Proceedings of the 18th Annual Hanford Life Sciences Symposium, Richland, Washington, October, 1978, Springfield, Virginia, Technical Information Center, US Department of Energy, pp. 132-146 (DOE Symposium Series 50, NTIS CONF-781016).

WAIBEL, R. (1975) [The effect of low frequency electric fields on man,] Graz, Austria, Technical University (Dissertation) (in German).

WALCOTT, C. (1974) The homing pigeons. Am. Sci., 62: 542-552.

WARE, B.J. (1975) Effect of 765 kV transmission lines on animal grazing habits, revised ed., American Electric Power Service Corporation.

WEIRICH, J., HOHNLOSER, S., ANTONI, H. (1983) Factors determining the susceptibility of the isolated guinea-pig heart to fibrillation induced by sinusoidal alternating current at frequencies from 1 - 1000 Hz. Basic Res. Cardiol., 78: 604-616.

WERTHEIMER, N. & LEEPER, E. (1979) Electrical wiring configurations and childhood cancer. Am. J. Epidemiol., 109: 273-284.

WERTHEIMER, N. & LEEPER, E. (1980) Letters to the editor; the author's reply. Am. J. Epidemiol., 112: 167-168.

WERTHEIMER, N. & LEEPER, E. (1982) Adult cancer related to electrical wires near the home. Int. J. Epidemiol., 11(4): 345-355.

WEVER, R. (1968) [Influence of weak electromagnetic fields on the circadian periodicity of man.] Naturwissenschaften, 55: 29 (in German, NASA translation, X68-182216).

WILSON, B.W., ANDERSON, L.E., HILTON, D.I., & PHILLIPS, R.D. (1981) Chronic exposure to 60 Hz electric fields: effects on pineal function in the rat. Bioelectromagnetics, 2: 371-380.

WILSON, B.W., ANDERSON, L.E., HILTON, D.I. & PHILLIPS, R.D. (1983) Erratum, chronic exposure to 60-Hz electric fields: Effects on pineal function in the rat. Bioelectromagnetics, 4: 293.

WRIGHT, W.E., PETERS, J.M., & MACK, T.M. (1982) Leukaemia in workers exposed to electrical and magnetic fields. Lancet, 11: 1160-1161.

ZAFFANELLA, L.E. & DENO, D.W. (1978) Electrostatic and electromagnetic effects of ultra-high-voltage transmission lines, Palo Alto, California, Electric Power Research Institute (Final report EPRI EL-802).

APPENDIX I

The electromagnetic environment in the home[a]

A. 60-Hz electric-field strengths at the centre of various rooms in a typical home in the USA in 1974

Room	V/m
Laundry room	0.8
Dining room	0.9
Bathroom	1.2 - 1.5
Kitchen	2.6
Bedrooms	2.4 - 7.8
Living room	3.3
Hallway	13.0

B. Typical values of electric-field strength (V/m) from 115-V, 60-Hz home appliances (USA) at 30 cm from source

Electric blanket	250[b]
Broiler	130
Stereo	90
Refrigerator	60
Electric iron	60
Hand mixer	50
Toaster	40
Hair Dryer	40
Colour TV	30
Coffee pot	30
Vacuum cleaner	16
Incadescent light bulb	2

C. Localized 60-Hz magnetic flux densities in the vicinity (a few cm) of some electric appliances (mT)

1 - 2.5
- 325 watt soldering gun
- Hair dryer

0.5 - 1.0
- Can opener
- Kitchen range
- Electric shaver
- Fluorescent desk lamp

0.1 - 0.5
- Colour TV
- Food mixer
- Electric drill

0.01 - 0.1
- Garbage disposal
- Clothes dryer
- Vacuum cleaner
- Electric toaster

APPENDIX I (contd).

D. Leakàge currents passing through the body to earth from household appliances (μA); the values should be compared to ANSI standards for fixed appliances (750 μA) and for cord-connected appliances (500 μA)

Coffee mill	380
Refrigerator	40
Sewing machine	34
Coffee pot	6

E. Induced currents flowing in the earthed arm of an 80-kg, 1.75-m human being with a heating pad or electric blanket in a representative location

Heating pad	18 μA
Electric blanket	7 - 27 μA

F. Typical values of measured dispersed ambient magnetic flux densities[c]

Location	Magnetic Flux Density (μT)
University of Pennsylvania Hospital	0.2 - 0.4; 60 Hz
Princeton Hospital	0.03 - 0.1; 60 Hz
Park Falls (Wisconsin) Hospital	0.05 - 0.8; 60 Hz
Industrial Plant, Park Falls (Wisconsin)	0.3 - 6; 60 Hz
Scientific Laboratory, Pensacola, Florida	0.5 - 1; 60 Hz
IIT Research Institute office areas	5; 60 Hz
Stamford (Conneticut) railroad station	2 - 20; 25 Hz
Private dwelling	0.1 - 10.1; 60 Hz

[a] From: Miller (1974), Bridges (1975), Sheppard & Eiisenbud (1977), Atoian (1978), Bridges & Preache (1981).
[b] Actual human exposure would be higher since the blanket would be at a distance of less than 30 cm.
[c] From: Miller (1974).

APPENDIX I REFERENCES

ATOIAN, G.E. (1978) Are there biological and psychological effects due to extra-high voltage installations? IEEE Trans. Power Appl. Syst., 97: 8-16.

BRIDGES, E.J. (1975) Biological effects of high-voltage electric fields, Palo Alto, California, Electric Power Research Institute, p. 206 (Field Report EPRI 381-1).

BRIDGES, J.E. & PREACHE, M. (1981) Biological influences of power frequency electric fields - a tutorial review from a physical and experimental viewpoint. Proc. IEEE, 69: 1092-1120.

MILLER, D.A. (1974) Electric and magnetic fields produced by commercial power systems. In: Llaurado, J., Sances, A., & Battocletti, J.H., ed. Biologic and clinical effects of low frequency magnetic and electric fields, Springfield, Illinois, Charles C. Thomas, pp. 62-70.

SHEPPARD, A.R. & EISENBUD, M. (1977) Biologic effects of electric and magnetic fields of extremely low frequency, New York, New York University Press.